Hepatitis C in Renal Disease, Hemodialysis and Transplantation

Contributions to Nephrology

Vol. 176

Series Editor

Claudio Ronco Vicenza

Hepatitis C in Renal Disease, Hemodialysis and Transplantation

Volume Editor

Jose M. Morales Madrid

Co-Editors

Beatriz Domínguez-Gil Madrid
Josep M. Campistol Barcelona
Michel Jadoul Brussels
Lionel Rostaing Toulouse
David Roth Miami, Fla.

9 figures and 8 tables, 2012

KARGER Basel · Freiburg · Paris · London · New York · New Delhi · Bangkok · Beijing · Tokyo · Kuala Lumpur · Singapore · Sydney

Contributions to Nephrology
(Founded 1975 by Geoffrey M. Berlyne)

Jose M. Morales
Instituto de Investigación
Hospital 12 de Octubre
ES-28001 Madrid

Library of Congress Cataloging-in-Publication Data

Hepatitis C in renal disease, hemodialysis and transplantation / volume editor, Jose M. Morales ; co-editors, Beatriz Domínguez-Gil ... [et al.].
p.; cm. -- (Contributions to nephrology, ISSN 0302-5144 ; v. 176)
Includes bibliographical references and indexes.
ISBN 978-3-8055-9820-0 (hard cover: alk. paper) -- ISBN 978-3-8055-9821-7 (e-ISBN)
I. Morales, Jose M. (Jose Maria), 1949- II. Domínguez-Gil, Beatriz. III. Series: Contributions to nephrology; v. 176. 0302-5144
[DNLM: 1. Hepatitis C. 2. Kidney Diseases--complications. 3. Kidney Transplantation. 4. Renal Dialysis. W1 CO778UN v.176 2012 / WC 536]
616.3'623--dc23

2011046047

Bibliographic Indices. This publication is listed in bibliographic services, including Current Contents® and Index Medicus.

www.karger.com
Printed in Germany on acid-free and non-aging paper (ISO 9706) by Bosch Druck, Ergolding
ISSN 0302–5144
e-ISSN 1662–2782
ISBN 978–3–8055–9820–0
e-ISBN 978–3–8055–9821–7

Contents

Preface

Hepatitis C virus (HCV) infection is a major health problem worldwide. According to the reports, there are currently over 150 million HCV-infected people on the five continents. Although important advances in the diagnosis, prevention and therapy of HCV infection have been made, in most countries, particularly in the developing countries, it remains an important health problem.

HCV infection has been considered as a systemic disease: not only does it affect the liver, it can induce autoimmune, dermatological and renal disease. Not surprisingly, soon after the discovery of HCV as the major cause of non-A non-B hepatitis, HCV infection was recognized as an important cause and consequence of chronic kidney disease. For these reasons, Kidney Disease Improving Global Outcomes (KDIGO) decided to include HCV infection as an important topic to develop in nephrology, dialysis and transplantation. The document elaborated by a group of experts: 'KDIGO clinical practice guidelines for the prevention, diagnosis, evaluation and treatment of hepatitis C in chronic kidney disease' [Kidney Int 2008;73(suppl 109):S1–S99] is the most important and complete contribution ever published on this topic.

Three years later after this publication, we had the initiative to review the most important recent news concerning HCV virus infection and nephrology, dialysis and transplantation. I personally contacted first Dr. Jadoul, Dr. Rostaing and Dr. Roth to start this project accepted by Karger Publishers as a new volume of *Contributions in Nephrology*. We have elaborated this publication including the most important topics concerning HCV infection, renal disease and problems with dialysis in the general population and also in renal transplant patients. We also included a chapter that discusses the emerging problem of renal complications associated with HCV virus in patients with HIV infection.

All international authors of this undertaking, most of them participants of KDIGO, are relevant investigators who have contributed to the knowledge of HCV infection in patients with chronic kidney disease. I acknowledge the important effort and contributions of all authors who made it all possible.

Particularly, I acknowledge the Co-Editors' enthusiasm with the project and criticism. Finally, I would like to express my gratitude to Karger Publishers for accepting our suggestion, to Novartis for their generous support and to my hospital and the Institute of Investigation of Hospital 12 de Octubre for their continuous stimulus.

Jose M. Morales, Madrid

Morales JM (ed): Hepatitis C in Renal Disease, Hemodialysis and Transplantation.
Contrib Nephrol. Basel, Karger, 2012, vol 176, pp 1–9

Hepatitis C: Epidemiology, Diagnosis, Natural History and Therapy

Stanislas Pol · Anaïs Vallet-Pichard · Marion Corouge · Vincent O. Mallet

Université Paris Descartes, APHP, Hôpital Cochin, Unité d'Hépatologie, INSERM U-1016, Institut Cochin, Paris, France

Abstract

With an estimated prevalence of 3% in the world population (around 170 million infected individuals worldwide), hepatitis C virus (HCV) heavily burdens public health. Even though the incidence of new infections is declining, at least in industrialized countries where they are mainly restricted to intravenous drug users, morbidity and mortality (which means also HCV-induced costs) associated with HCV infection are expected to increase over the next decade. Models suggest that the incidence of hepatocellular carcinoma and HCV-related mortality will still increase until about 2015. The prevalence of the disease, the risk of progression of fibrosis to cirrhosis or hepatocellular carcinoma, mainly but not only in patients with liver comorbidities such as metabolic syndrome and/or heavy alcohol intake, evidences: (1) the need for a screening of chronic HCV infection as defined by both anti-HCV antibodies and detectable HCV RNA, (2) the evaluation of the extrahepatic (cryoglobulinemia-related vasculitis) or liver impact of chronic infection (by liver biopsy or noninvasive markers of fibrosis) and (3) the discussion of an antiviral treatment which is mainly the combination of pegylated interferon (one weekly subcutaneous injection) and ribavirin, a nucleosidic analogue with a twice daily oral intake. This 'standard of care' results in a mean of 60% of sustained virologic response corresponding to viral eradication, which allows the inactivation of necroinflammation and the remodeling of fibrosis. New antiviral treatments (direct-acting antivirals like protease NS3/4, polymerase NS5B, NS5A, entry inhibitors or other drugs like cyclophilin inhibitors, new interferons, immune modulators or therapeutic vaccine) are being rapidly developed (the approval of the first generation protease inhibitors is expected for spring 2011). The next step appears to be the combination of these oral drugs allowing a better safety and efficacy of the treatment.

With an estimated prevalence of 3% in the world population (around 170 million infected individuals worldwide), hepatitis C virus (HCV) heavily burdens public health [1, 2]. Even though the incidence of new infections is declining, at least in industrialized countries where they are mainly restricted to intravenous drug users, morbidity and mortality (which means also HCV-induced costs) associated with HCV infection are expected to increase over the next decade. Models suggest that the incidence of hepatocellular carcinoma (HCC) and HCV-related mortality will still increase until about 2015. The prevalence of the disease, the risk of progression of fibrosis to cirrhosis or HCC, mainly but not only in patients with liver comorbidities such as metabolic syndrome and/or heavy alcohol intake, evidences: (1) the need for a screening of chronic HCV infection as defined by both anti-HCV antibodies and detectable HCV RNA, (2) the evaluation of both the extrahepatic (cryoglobulinemia-associated vasculitis) and liver impact of chronic infection (by liver biopsy or noninvasive markers of fibrosis) and (3) the discussion of an antiviral treatment which is mainly based in 2011 on the combination of pegylated interferon and ribavirin (RBV; genotypes 2–6) or on a triple therapy combining protease inhibitors of HCV (telaprevir and boceprevir), pegylated interferon and RBV (genotypes 1).

Epidemiology and Diagnosis of HCV Infection

HCV infection is one of the main causes of chronic liver disease worldwide [1]. The estimated prevalence of 3% in the world population heavily burdens public health [1, 2]. In Western Europe, HCV prevalence ranges from 0.4 to 3% [3]. Prevalence is higher in Eastern Europe and the Middle East, up to 13% in Egypt [4]. Thus, the number of chronically infected patients may exceed 170 millions, but most of them have no knowledge of their infection. The total HCV-infected population in the US was estimated to decline from 3.15 million in 2005 to 2.47 million in 2021 as disease burden increased as the infected population aged. During the same period, the mortality rate is expected to increase from 2.0 to 2.9%. The diagnosed population was 50% of the total infections, while less than 4% of the total infections were treated.

The risk of HCV contamination is almost only parenteral: before the 1990s, the main routes of transmission were blood product transfusion, intravenous drug use or unsafe injection procedures accounting for approximately 70% of cases in industrialized countries. Since the systematic screening of blood products, the residual risk of transfusion HCV infection is extremely low (around 1/2,000,000). Currently in industrialized countries, the routes of transmission remain intravenous or nasal drug use, mother to child transmission (about 5–10%) and unsafe medical or surgical procedures. The risk of heterosexual transmission is low, but high in human immunodeficiency virus (HIV)-infected men who have sex with men [5]. The dialysis-related risk is known (around 2%/

year), varying according to the countries: health care-related transmission can be eradicated with a strict respect of hygiene rules [6]. Occasional transmissions are also observed due to tattooing or acupuncture with unsafe materials, and about 30% of hepatitis C infections remain unexplained.

Six HCV genotypes and a large number of subtypes (from a to f) are known, and some of them have spread throughout the world. Genotype 1 (subtypes 1a and 1b) is the most prevalent genotype worldwide: genotype 1b is highly prevalent in Japan and Europe and genotype 1a in the US. Genotype 2 is observed in clusters in the Mediterranean region. Genotype 3a is frequent in the Indian subcontinent and in European intravenous drug abusers [3]. Genotype 4 is historically described in Egypt and Africa, but its prevalence and its incidence increase in European intravenous drug users. Finally genotypes 5 are more rarely found, and genotypes 6 are mainly observed in south China [7].

The diagnosis of HCV infection is based on the detection of anti-HCV antibodies by third-generation ELISA assays. The distinction between resolved infection and chronic infection is only based on the detection (active infection) or not (recovery) of the HCV RNA in the serum by using sensitive molecular assays. The threshold of these procedures is around 15 IU/ml. Chronic HCV infection should be proven by the presence of both anti-HCV and HCV RNA [8].

Natural History of HCV Infection

About 10% of acute hepatitis cases are related to acute HCV infection in Europe. Because of systematic screening of blood products, strict respect of hygiene rules and increased efficacy of treatment of chronic HCV infection, the incidence of acute HCV infection has decreased, and is now about 1/100,000 subjects per year. But this rate is probably underestimated due to large numbers of asymptomatic forms (50–90% of cases). Spontaneous resolution of acute hepatitis occurs in around 30% of cases [9], according to the route of transmission, the presence of symptomatic hepatitis, the age at which infection occurred and immune status. Recently, polymorphisms of the IL28B (CC, TT, CT), a gene located near the lambda interferon gene, were associated with the rates of spontaneous clearance of acute HCV hepatitis [10]: the CC genotype is clearly associated with a higher rate of spontaneous recovery and, interestingly, with fibrosis progression and a higher rate of sustained virologic response (SVR) under antiviral therapy.

Chronic infection is associated with variable degrees of hepatic inflammation and fibrosis progression, regardless of HCV genotype and viral load. The long-term hepatic impact of HCV infection is highly variable, from minimal changes to chronic hepatitis, extensive fibrosis, and cirrhosis, with or without HCC. Fibrosis progression takes several decades and is associated with cofactors such as alcohol consumption, tobacco or cannabis smoking, metabolic syndrome or

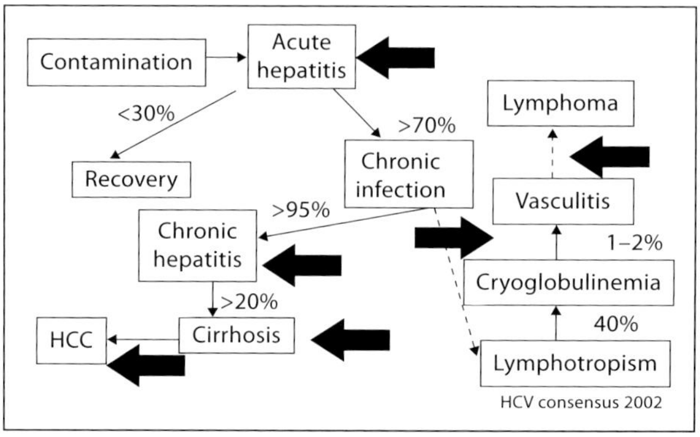

Fig. 1. Times for treatment of HCV infection during the natural history are indicated by the arrow. Treatment duration depends on genotypes and viral kinetics.

diabetes mellitus (to which HCV itself predisposes), older age of acquisition, HIV coinfection or coinfection with other hepatotropic viruses. According to the presence of cofactors, between 10 and 40% of patients will develop cirrhosis [11]. HCC occurs at an estimated incidence of 3% per year in cirrhotic patients and incidence of death related to complications of cirrhosis is about 4% per year. Patients diagnosed with HCC have a 33% probability of death during the first year [12].

Diagnosis of active chronic HCV infection (anti-HCV positivity and HCV RNA positivity since more than 6 months) necessitates the evaluation of both the hepatic and extrahepatic impact (cryoglobulinemia-associated vasculitis) of chronic infection. The evaluation of the liver impact of hepatitis (stage and grade) is based either on liver biopsy or on noninvasive tests. The concordance between the biochemical (Fibrotest, Fibrometre, Hepascore, Forns index, Fib-4. . .) or morphological (elastometry by the Fibroscan which evaluates the liver stiffness) tests, may avoid around a half of liver biopsy. The main advantage of these noninvasive tests is to allow the yearly follow-up of fibrosis in untreated patients.

Treatment of HCV Infection

The treatment is recommended at any stage of HCV infection. At the acute phase, if HCV RNA is still detectable after a mean of 12 weeks, there is an indication for a 24-week course of pegylated interferon (PEGIFN) (associated with ribavirin (RBV) in HIV coinfected patients; fig. 1). If HCV RNA remains detectable at week 4 or week 12, treatment duration should be prolonged to 48 weeks. At the chronic phase, antiviral therapy may be considered in any patient according to the recent EASL clinical practical guidelines [8]. We recommend treating patients with a significant impact of the chronic HCV infection (chronic fatigue, chronic hepatitis with necroinflammation and/or fibrosis >1 according to the Metavir scale) or symptomatic extrahepatic disease, mainly related to cryoglobulinemia-associated vasculitis with renal (membranoproliferative glomerulonephritis), cutaneous (purpura), neurologic (peripheric neuropathy) or rheumatologic complications (arthritis). Indeed, therapeutic progress is expected over the next 5 years, and all the treatments are associated with side effects, usually minor and manageable for the more frequent but sometimes severe for the less frequent (ophthalmologic, autoimmunity induction, acute psychiatric troubles. . .).

Recommended Therapy

The currently recommended therapy for chronic hepatitis C is a combination of PEG-IFN and RBV for 24 (genotypes 2 and 3) to 48 weeks (genotype 1), depending on the viral genotype and the immunologic status of the patient. Combination therapy allows for SVR in ~50% of patients, depending on host and viral characteristics, especially the viral genotype [13–15]. SVR is achieved in around 45% of genotype 1-infected patients treated for 48 weeks. SVR rates for patients with the less common genotypes 2 and 3 (and 5 or 6 probably while evidence is lower) are 76–85% when treated for 24 weeks. Treatment response to genotype 4 lies somewhere between that seen for genotype 1 and those of genotypes 2 and 3 [16]: 36 weeks of treatment may be as effective as 48 weeks for genotype 4-infected patients [16].

Serum concentration of HCV RNA at the time of initiation of antiviral therapy is another determinant of outcome. Sustained response rates are consistently higher in patients with low baseline HCV RNA levels, usually defined as <800,000 IU/ml [13–15]. Host factors also affect the chance of SVR, albeit less so than the genotype (except the IL28B polymorphism) [10]. They include age, race (according to different repartition of the IL28B polymorphisms according to ethnicity: African-Americans have lower response rate than Caucasians), gender, obesity, degree of hepatic fibrosis, and immunodepression.

Predicting Response to HCV Therapy

Responses to treatment are characterized by different viral kinetic profiles. Patients who achieve SVR have typically a rapid initial decline in viral level (early virologic response or EVR). EVR reflects the efficiency of suppression of replication, followed by a second, slower phase of decline in viral load until undetectable levels of circulating virus are achieved. The second phase is believed to be due to clearance of virus-infected cells. EVR is classically defined by a 99% or greater decrease in HCV RNA at 12 weeks of antiviral therapy: complete EVR (cEVR) by an HCV RNA undetectable at 12 weeks and partial EVR (pEVR) by a 99% decrease in HCV RNA level at 12 weeks with a PCR remaining positive. cEVR has a positive predictive value (PPV) of 72% for SVR

[13, 17]. Patients with pEVR are less likely to achieve SVR (PPV of 21%) than patients who have undetectable HCV RNA at 12 weeks (PPV of 84%). In genotype 1-infected patients, treatment must be discontinued in patients who do not achieve a 99% decrease in HCV RNA at 12 weeks and in all cases if the 24-week PCR remains positive (the likelihood of achieving SVR is about 1%). Patients with pEVR and those with negative 24-week PCR will be treated for 72 weeks. In genotype 3-infected patients, treatment duration is longer (48 weeks) if they do not achieve a cEVR. Genotype 2-infected patients always achieve a cEVR. Rapid viral response (RVR), defined as a negative qualitative PCR assay at week 4, has a high PPV of SVR ranging around 90% in mono-infected patients and 82% in coinfected patients. According to the early viral kinetics (RVR, cEVR or the so-called eRVR, extended RVR corresponding to undetectability of HCV RNA at both week 4 and week 12 of therapy), treatment duration may be shortened or prolonged.

Tailoring Anti-HCV Therapy

In genotype 1-infected patients who do not achieve an RVR, the benefit of a longer duration (72 weeks) remains debated. In the peculiar subgroup of patients with a negative PCR at week 4 (and mainly in those with a pretreatment baseline viral load below 250,000 IU/ml) the SVR rate is high (92%), despite a short course of only 24 weeks of therapy [18]. In genotype 2- or 3-infected patients with a negative qualitative PCR at week 4, a reduction in the treatment duration to 12–16 weeks may be discussed if the doses of RBV are weight adjusted (around 15 mg/kg/day) and not fixed (800 mg/day).

Increasing the dose of PEG-IFN has not been proven to be effective in nonresponders, relapsers and naive patients. The dose-effect of RBV is suggested by pivotal studies reporting a dose effect of RBV for doses >10.6 mg/kg/day, with a direct relation between the received dose and SVR [19] and by a recent study which compared standard doses to high doses which were allowed by erythropoietin (EPO)-associated therapy [20]. Altogether, these studies suggest that, according to the genotype, the baseline viral load, and the early viral kinetics, the treatment dose and the treatment duration should be modulated to improve the SVR rate and reduce the rate of side effects. The recent EASL CPGs recommend a dose of 15 mg/kg/day in genotype 1–4-infected patients and a fixed dose of 800 mg/day in genotype 2–3-infected patients [8] but higher doses of RBV may allow to reduce the duration of therapy in these so-called easy to treat patients (12–16 weeks instead of 24 weeks) or to increase SVR in those with baseline negative predictors (high viral load, metabolic syndrome, extensive fibrosis or cirrhosis).

The Next Future of HCV Therapy

The treatment of HCV infection by a combination of pegylated interferon and RBV, according to early viral kinetics, leads to an SVR in more than 50% of patients with chronic infection. This SVR is a complete recovery of the infection (virologic recovery and fibrosis remodeling in the absence of liver comorbidities) [21–23] but more than 50% of genotype 1-infected patients do not achieve SVR. A better understanding of the viral cycle, and the characterization of viral enzymes which are potential targets, resulted in the development of new molecules, direct-acting antiviral drugs targeted against HCV, either specific of genotype 1 (NS3/NS4A protease inhibitors and NS5B polymerase inhibitors) or with a wider spectrum (NS5A or entry inhibitors), and nonspecific antivirals (new interferons, cyclophilin inhibitors).

The results of phase II and III trials of the first-generation (first wave) of protease inhibitors (telaprevir and boceprevir) have clearly demonstrated a 20–30% increase in the SVR rate of genotype 1-infected patients. Around 75% of genotype1-infected naïve patients achieved SVR with 12 weeks of triple therapy with Telaprevir and an overall treatment duration of 24 weeks (allowed in two thirds of patients who achieved an extended rapid virologic response, eRVR, defined as HCV RNA undetectability after 4 and 12 weeks of triple therapy) [20, 24, 25]; SVR was also achieved in around 65% of the same patients who were given 24–44 weeks of triple therapy with Boceprevir and the standard combination after a 4-week course of lead-in phase by the standard combination [26]. In treatment-experienced genotype 1-infected patients, the triple therapy allows around 85% of SVR in previous relapsers, 55% in previous partial responders and 30% in previous null responders [27, 28]. These new drugs have been approved in 2011, after a temporary approval for compassionate use in some countries for cirrhotic genotype 1 patients with previous relapse or partial response to the combination therapy. In the future, the main limitations of triple therapy will be safety (cutaneous rash or anemia which may be controlled), cost, compliance, viral resistance, and drug interactions that must be avoided by educating patients and physicians.

New strategies, including new IFNs [consensus IFN (alphacon-1) and λ-IFN], internal ribosomal entry site inhibitors, nucleosidic and nonnucleosidic polymerase inhibitors, interfering mRNAs, and therapeutic vaccines are under development.

The combination of the different new oral antiviral drugs with different viral targets for a duration of 24 weeks appears to be able to achieve a complete recovery (SVR) in HCV-infected patients, including null responders, and this is probably the next step in the improvement of the care and recovery of these patients. A better therapeutic schedule remains to be defined in patients with renal failure, including hemodialysis or renal transplantation, and data regarding the new drugs used in these patients, which apparently do not require dose adjustments to the renal function, are not available.

References

1 Shepard CW, Finelli L, Alter MJ: Global epidemiology of hepatitis C virus infection. Lancet Infect Dis 2005;5:558–567.
2 Lavanchy D: The global burden of hepatitis C. Liver Int 2009;29:74–81.
3 Esteban JI, Sauleda S, Quer J: The changing epidemiology of hepatitis C virus infection in Europe. J Hepatol 2008, 48:148–62.
4 Kamal SM, Nasser IA: Hepatitis C genotype 4: what we know what we don't yet know. Hepatology 2008;47:1371–1383.
5 van de Laar TJW, Matthews GV, Prins M, et al: Acute hepatitis C in HIV-infected men who have sex with men: an emerging sexually transmitted infection. AIDS 2010;24:1799–1812.
6 Jadoul M, Cornu C, van Ypersele de Strihou C: Universal precautions prevent hepatitis C virus transmission: a 54 month follow-up of the Belgian Multicenter Study. The Universitaires Cliniques St-Luc (UCL) Collaborative Group. Kidney Int 1998;53:1022–1025.
7 Antaki N, Craxi A, Kamal S, Moucari R, Van de Merwe S, Haffar S, et al: The neglected hepatitis C virus genotypes 4, 5 and 6: an international consensus report. Liver Int 2010;30:342–355.
8 EASL Clinical Practice Guidelines: Management of Hepatitis C virus infection. J Hepatol August 2011;55:245–264.
9 Santantonio T, Wiegang J, Gerlac JT: Acute hepatitis C: current status and remaining challenges. J Hepatol 2008;49:625–633.
10 Thomas DL, Thio CL, Martin MP, et al: Genetic variation in IL28B and spontaneous clearance of hepatitis C virus. Nature 2009;461:798–801.
11 Afdhal NH: The natural history of hepatitis C. Semin Liver Dis 2004;24:3–8.
12 Yang YD, Roberts LR: Hepatocellular carcinoma: a global view. Nat Rev Gastroenterol Hepatol 2010;7:448–458.
13 Manns MP, McHutchison JG, Gordon SC, et al: Peginterferon alfa-2b plus ribavirin compared with interferon alfa-2b plus ribavirin for initial treatment of chronic hepatitis C: a randomised trial. Lancet 2001;358:958–965.
14 Fried MW, Shiffman ML, Reddy KR, et al: Peginterferon alfa-2a plus ribavirin for chronic hepatitis C virus infection. N Engl J Med 2002;347:975–982.
15 Hadziyannis SJ, Sette H Jr, Morgan TR, et al: Peginterferon-alpha2a and ribavirin combination therapy in chronic hepatitis C: a randomized study of treatment duration and ribavirin dose. Ann Intern Med 2004;140:346–355.
16 Kamal S, El Tawil AA, Nakano T, et al: Peginterferon alpha-2b and ribavirin therapy in chronic hepatitis C genotype 4: impact of treatment duration and viral kinetics on sustained virological response. Gut 2005;54:858–866.
17 Davis GL, Wong JB, McHutchison JG, et al: Early virologic response to treatment with peginterferon alfa-2b plus ribavirin in patients with chronic hepatitis C. Hepatology 2003;38:645–652.
18 Zeuzem S, Buti M, Ferenci P, et al: Efficacy of 24 weeks treatment with peginterferon alfa-2b plus ribavirin in patients with chronic hepatitis C infected with genotype 1 and low pretreatment viremia. J Hepatol 2006;44:97–103.
19 Reddy KR, Hadziyannis SJ, Diago M, et al: The influence of cumulative peginterferon alpha-2a (40 kDa) and ribavirin (RBV) exposure on sustained virological response (SVR) rates in patients with genotype 1 chronic hepatitis C. J Hepatol 2005;42:217–217.
20 Shiffman ML, Salvatore J, Hubbard S, et al: Treatment of chronic hepatitis C virus genotype 1 with peginterferon, ribavirin, and epoetin alpha. Hepatology 2007;46:371–379.
21 Fontaine H, Chaix ML, Lagneau JL, et al: Recovery from hepatitis C in long-term responders to ribavirin plus interferon alfa. Lancet 2000;356:41.
22 Poynard T, McHutchison J, Davis GL, Esteban-Mur R, Goodman Z, Bedossa P, et al: Impact of interferon α-2b and ribavirin on progression of liver fibrosis in patients with chronic hepatitis C. Hepatology 2000;32:1131–1137.

23 Mallet V, Gilgenkrantz H, Serpaggi J, Verkarre V, Vallet-Pichard A, Fontaine H, et al: The relationship of regression of cirrhosis to outcome in chronic hepatitis C. Ann Intern Med 2008;149:399–403.
24 Mc Hutchison JG, Everson GT, Gordon SC, et al: Telaprevir with peginterferon and ribavirin for chronic HCV genotype 1 infection. N Engl J Med 2009;360:1827–1838.
25 Hezode C, Forestier N, Dusheiko G, et al: Telaprevir and peginterferon with or without ribavirin for chronic HCV genotype 1 infection. N Engl J Med 2009;360:1839–1850.
26 Kwo PY, Lawitz EJ, McCone J, et al: Efficacy of boceprevir, an NS3 protease inhibitor, in combination with peginterferon alpha-2b and ribavirin in treatment-naïve patients with genotype 1 hepatitis C infection (SPRINT-1): an open-label, randomised, multicentre phase 2 trial. Lancet 2010;376:705–716.
27 McHutchison JG, Manns MP, Muir AJ, et al: Telaprevir for previously treated chronic HCV infection. N Engl J Med 2010;362:1292–303.
28 Bacon BR, Gordon SC, Lawitz E, Marcellin P, Vierling JM, Zeuzem S, et al: Boceprevir for previously treated chronic HCV genotype 1 infection. N Engl J Med 2011;364:1207–1217.

Stanislas Pol, MD, PhD
APHP, Hôpital Cochin, Hépatologie
27 rue du faubourg Saint Jacques
FR–75014 Paris (France)
Tel. +33 0 1 58 41 30 00, E-Mail stanislas.pol@cch.aphp.fr

Morales JM (ed): Hepatitis C in Renal Disease, Hemodialysis and Transplantation.
Contrib Nephrol. Basel, Karger, 2012, vol 176, pp 10–23

Hepatitis C and Renal Disease: Epidemiology, Diagnosis, Pathogenesis and Therapy

Jose M. Morales[a] · N. Kamar[b,c] · L. Rostaing[b,c]

[a]Department of Nephrology, Hospital 12 de Octubre, Madrid, Spain; [b]Department of Nephrology, Dialysis, and Organ Transplantation, CHU Rangueil, [c]INSERM U563, IFR-30, Toulouse, France

Abstract

There is an increased evidence for the association between hepatitis C virus (HCV) infection and kidney diseases. Recent epidemiological studies strongly suggest that HCV infection is a risk factor for proteinuria and/or impaired renal function. Type I membranoproliferative glomerulonephritis (MPGN) associated with type II cryoglobulinemia is the most frequent renal disease, and non-cryoglobulinemic MPGN and membranous glomerulonephritis are less frequently associated with active HCV infection. The pathogenesis of these lesions are related to the deposition of immune complexes in the glomeruli, and recently it has been described that toll-like receptor 3 could have a pathogenic role establishing a link between viral infection and glomerulonephritis. Patients with HCV-related glomerulopathies should be treated with angiotensin-converting enzyme inhibitors in association or not with angiotensin receptor blockers, as well as with anti-HCV therapy. The latter relies on a combined antiviral therapy of standard or pegylated interferon-α and ribavirin. We recommend the treatment of patients for at least 48 weeks, and the continuation of antiviral therapy, even in the absence of a decrease in HCV RNA concentration of 2-log at week 12. Ribavirin doses should be adapted according to creatinine clearance in order to avoid its main side effect, i.e. hemolytic anemia. Combined antiviral therapy and immunosuppression (cyclophosphamide or rituximab with steroids) may be the treatment of choice for patients with severe renal disease, i.e. nephrotic syndrome and/or progressive renal failure, or diseases that are refractory to anti-HCV therapy alone.

Patients with hepatitis C virus (HCV) infection can develop chronic hepatitis, liver cirrhosis and hepatocellular carcinoma. Several extrahepatic complications have also been associated with HCV infection, including hematological, dermatologic, autoimmune and kidney diseases [1]. There is an increasing evidence for the association between HCV infection and glomerular disease in both native and transplanted kidneys [2, 3]. Type I membranoproliferative glomerulonephritis (MPGN) associated with type II cryoglobulinemia is the more frequent renal disease, and non-cryoglobulinemic MPGN and membranous glomerulonephritis (MGN) are less frequently described to be associated with HCV infection [2–4].

In this chapter, we will review the literature concerning the increased risk of chronic kidney disease (CKD) in HCV-positive patients, the most important kidney diseases associated with HCV infection as well as their clinical manifestations, pathogenesis and therapy.

Epidemiology of Chronic Kidney Disease in Patients with HCV Infection

HCV-infected patients, including those with kidney or liver transplants, have an increased risk of glomerular lesions leading to CKD. These alterations have been described in the presence or absence of significant liver disease: however, all patients with HCV-associated GN are HCV RNA positive in the serum [2–4].

Fabrizi et al. [5] reported that the prevalence of HCV seropositivity in case series of patients with MPGN is about 10 times greater than the reported prevalence in HCV-negative patients. This elevated prevalence of MPGN comparing general population was also described in both live and autopsy series [6, 7]. Recently, several epidemiologic studies reporting CKD prevalence and its clinical significance in patients with HCV infection have been described. In a study from the US, 18,002 patients with HCV infection were identified and compared with 25,137 controls with estimated glomerular filtration rate (eGFR) >60 ml/m/1.73 m^2 at baseline [8]. Notably, HCV infection was associated with a higher risk of developing CKD stages 3–5. As expected, increasing age, hypertension and diabetes were associated with significantly higher risks of developing CKD in HCV-positive patients and controls. Decompensated liver disease was a strong predictor of CKD in both groups and, remarkably, HCV-infected patients had a shorter time to CKD. Although information of proteinuria was absent, this study clearly demonstrated that HCV infection is associated with higher risk and shorter time to CKD. In another study, 552 anti-HCV-positive patients were compared with 313 HCV-negative patients. CKD was defined as eGFR <60 ml/m/1.73 m^2 and/or persistence of proteinuria >6 months on urine analysis by dipstick. The prevalence of CKD was significantly higher in HCV patients (9.6 vs. 5.1%), and these patients showed a shorter time to develop CKD and end-stage renal disease. Interestingly, a higher baseline viral load was an independent predictor of CKD [9].

A cross-sectional analysis of the NHANES III data demonstrated an age-dependent association between HCV seropositivity and albuminuria (adjusted odds ratio of 1.84 for ages 40–59 years and 1.27 for ages ≥60 years) [10]. In the ≥60 years group, 46% of HCV-positive individuals had albuminuria compared with 24% of those who where HCV antibody negative. However, this study found no significant association between HCV seropositivity and low estimated GFR. In a cross-sectional analysis from Taiwan, non-diabetic patients who were anti-HCV positive had a high prevalence of proteinuria (>1 positive dipstick) than the seronegative group (8.3 vs. 5.1%, p = 0.002) [11]. In multivariable analysis, the association between HCV status and proteinuria had an odds ratio of 1.84, although there was no association with low eGFR.

In a study from Italy in 320 predialysis patients, the incidence of HCV infection was 6.25%, which is much higher than that expected for Europe, i.e. 0.2–3.5% [12]. As an example of this geographic variation, authors from Norway including a prospective cohort study of 1,010 HCV-positive patients diagnosed between 1990 and 2000, demonstrated that renal failure caused by MPGN occurred in 0.2% [13]. Therefore, all these data described above strongly suggest that HCV infection is a risk factor for proteinuria and/or impaired renal function.

The main clinical manifestations of glomerular disease in HCV-positive patients are the presence of proteinuria and microscopic hematuria with or without impaired kidney function [2]. Therefore, it has been recommended by international guidelines that HCV-infected patients be tested at least annually for proteinuria, hematuria and eGFR [3]. This is especially important particularly in patients with cryoglobulinemia. Guidelines also recommended that a kidney biopsy be performed in HCV-infected patients with clinical evidence of glomerulonephritis (GN) [3]. Early diagnosis and therapy of HCV-associated GN may improve clinical outcomes [4].

Diagnosis of Glomerular Diseases Associated with HCV Infection

Mixed Cryoglobulinemia and Cryoglobulinemic Glomerulonephritis

Clinical and Laboratory Findings

HCV infection is the major cause of mixed cryoglobulinemia (MC), a systemic vasculitis characterized by arthralgias, arthritis, Raynaud phenomena, purpura, peripheral neuropathy, hypocomplementemia and kidney disease.

The presence of cryoglobulins is essential for the diagnosis, and usually HCV RNA is present in the serum [14, 15]. Hypocomplementemia and positive rheumatoid factor can also be observed. Some patients exhibited normal or only mild elevation of liver enzyme values. Clinical manifestations of kidney disease include nephrotic or non-nephrotic proteinuria, hematuria and variable degrees of reduced eGFR. Notably, acute nephritic syndrome or nephrotic syndrome can be the clinical presentation in 25 and 20% of these patients, respectively. Clinical signs of MC, such as purpura, arthralgias or neuropathy, can precede in several years the presence of kidney disease [14, 15].

HCV infection is mainly associated with type II MC, and type I MPGN, also called cryoglobulinemic GN, is the more frequent kidney lesion.

Pathology

Cryoglobulinemic GN typically includes evidence of immune complex deposition in the glomeruli and changes of type I MPGN. On light microscopy, glomeruli may demonstrate prominent hypercellularity as a result of massive infiltration of glomerular capillaries with mononuclear and polymorphonuclear leukocytes. Glomeruli show accentuation of lobulation of the tuft architecture, and may have a combination of increased matrix and mesangial cells, capillary endothelial swelling, splitting of capillary basement membrane, intracapillary thrombi and accumulation of eosinophilic material representing precipitated immune complexes or cryoglobulins. Vasculitis of the small and medium-sized renal arteries can also be present. Immunofluorescence usually demonstrates deposition of IgM, IgG and C3 in the mesangium and capillary walls. Subendothelial immune complexes are usually observed on electron microscopy and may also have a fibrillar or immunotactoid pattern suggestive of cryoglobulin deposits [3, 14, 15].

Clinicopathological Correlation

The presence of massive intraluminal thrombi, vasculitis or both is more commonly observed in patients with acute nephritic syndrome and rapid progression to kidney failure. Exsudative or lobular MPGN are associated with nephrotic and/or nephritic syndrome, whereas mesangioproliferative GN is associated with proteinuria and microscopic hematuria with normal renal function [3].

Outcome

Clinical course is variable; in the majority of patients, renal disease slowly progresses but does not progress to kidney failure in spite of the presence of proteinuria and some degree of renal impairment. Even some patients with cryoglobulinemic MPGN with massive thrombi and vasculitis can spontaneously reverse. Risk factors to develop end-stage renal disease are: older age, recurrent purpura, elevated cryocrit, hypocomplementemia and high serum creatinine at diagnosis [2, 3].

Non-Cryoglobulinemic Membranoproliferative Glomerulonephritis

Some patients with HCV infection can develop MPGN without exhibited cryoglobulins in the serum. The clinical picture, pathologic findings and laboratory data characteristically are indistinguishable from idiopathic type I MPGN except the presence of HCV antibodies and HCV RNA in the serum [2]. On electron microscopy, subendothelial and mesangial immune complexes can be detected without a distinctive substructure.

Membranous Glomerulonephritis

MGN is also associated with HCV infection. Clinical manifestations, outcome and pathology are similar to those of idiopathic MGN. All patients have serum HCV RNA-positive status accompanied by normal serum complement and negative cryoglobulins and rheumatoid factor [2–4, 16]. The characteristic finding on light microscopy is a diffuse thickening of the glomerular basement membrane without mesangial proliferation. The immunofluorescence demonstrates diffuse and granular deposits of IgG, C3 and IgA. Electron microscopy identifies diffuse subepithelial immune deposits.

Other Glomerular Diseases

Occasionally, other glomerular lesions in HCV-positive patients are reported including acute proliferative GN, focal segmental glomerulosclerosis, rapidly progressive GN, IgA nephropathy, thrombotic microangiopathy, fibrillary GN and immunotactoid glomerulopathy [3].

Pathogenesis of Glomerulonephritis Associated with HCV Infection

The pathogenesis of cryoglobulinemic GN associated with HCV infection is related to the deposition of immune complexes containing HCV proteins, anti-HCV antibodies and rheumatoid factor IgM with activity anti-IgG [17]. Viral antigens have been detected by immunohistochemistry [18] and by in situ hybridization [19]. Also, laser microdissection is a useful method for measuring HCV RNA genomic sequences of HCV core protein in glomeruli and tubules in patients with HCV-related GN [20]. On the other hand, the disappearance of proteinuria after interferon (IFN) therapy with elimination of HCV RNA in the serum strongly suggests the pathogenic role of HCV in this type of GN.

Recently, it has been described that toll-like receptor 3 (TLR3) messenger RNA expression was elevated in mesangial cells in HCV-associated GN and was associated with enhanced proinflammatory cytokines [21].This finding has been corroborated in a study from Egypt demonstrating that TLR3 expression was significantly higher in patients with HCV-positive GN than in HCV-negative patients and controls. Also, TLR3 expression correlated positively with HCV viral load, interleukin-1β and impaired renal function in patients with HCV-associated GN. In summary, TLR3 expression is upregulated in patients with HCV-associated GN, and overexpression is associated with reduced renal function and increased interleukin-1β level [22]. Another study suggests a novel role for IFN-γ-inducible protein and TNF-α in HCV-associated GN [23]. Therefore, these studies suggest a role of TLR3 in HCV-associated GN that could establish a link between viral infection and GN.

In patients with non-cryoglobulinemic MPGN associated with HCV infection, pathogenesis may be related to the deposition of immune complexes, HCV antigens and IgG antibodies (anti-HCV) in the glomeruli similar to immune complexes in GN associated with hepatitis B virus infection [2].

The pathogenesis of MGN in HCV-infected patients may be related to the deposition of immune complexes containing HCV proteins in the glomerular basement membrane. In spite of viral antigens that have been detected by methods mentioned before and the findings that IFN therapy may improve proteinuria, there is no consensus about the real pathogenetic role of HCV in this type of GN [2, 3].

Treatment of Glomerular Lesions Associated with HCV Infection

Cryoglobulinemic membranoproliferative GN is the most frequent HCV-related renal injury. Renal disease is the first cause of morbidity and mortality in MC patients. Hence, even if the HCV-related liver injury is not an indication for antiviral therapy, HCV-related renal disease requires a specific treatment. This treatment relies on either anti-HCV therapy alone in cases of moderate renal disease, or on combined antiviral and immunosuppressive therapies in cases of severe renal disease, i.e. nephrotic syndrome and/or progressive renal failure, or conditions that are refractory to anti-HCV therapy alone.

Symptomatic Therapy

Blood pressure control, diuretics, the blockade of the renin-angiotensin system using either angiotensin-converting enzyme inhibitors (ACEIs) alone or combined with angiotensin receptor blockers (ARBs), as well as the treatment of hyperlipidemia, are of proven benefit.

Anti-HCV Therapy

Because a link has been established between HCV infection and the occurrence of cryoglobulinemic MPGN, antiviral therapies have been used in HCV-positive patients presenting with GN in order to achieve clearance of HCV from the serum and, consequently, to have a beneficial effect on renal injury.

The AASLD (American Association for the Study of Liver Diseases) has published guidelines for the CKD population stating that 'when HCV infection is identified in persons with CKD, IFN-based antiviral treatment must be considered, but the regimen will vary depending of the kidney disease (. . .). The decision to treat must take into account the competing severities of the CKD and the chronic liver disease, the risks of the treatment itself (. . .), and whether there are comorbid conditions that may affect morbidity and mortality, such as cardiovascular disease' [24]. The kidneys play a major role in the catabolism and filtration of both IFN and ribavirin; thus, their clearances may be affected in subjects with CKD. The clearance of pegylated IFN (peg-IFN) is affected in those with CKD, although hemodialysis does not affect its clearance. Hence, the AASLD guidelines recommend subcutaneous weekly doses of 1 μg/kg of peg-α2b-IFN and of 135 μg of peg-α2a-IFN to patients with stage 3–5 CKD [24]. Because ribavirin is eliminated by the kidney, and if overdosed might result in dramatic anemia, ribavirin therapy is contraindicated when creatinine clearance is <50 ml/min. Hence, most data regarding HCV treatment in the CKD population deal with the use of either standard α-IFN or peg-α-IFN.

Interferon-α

In the early 1990s, standard IFN-α was used alone at different doses, i.e. 3–10 MU three times a week: unfortunately, the results were disappointing. In 15 patients who had a complete clearance of HCV RNA after IFN-α therapy, an improvement in renal function was observed [25]. However, there was no effect on proteinuria, and all patients relapsed. IFN-α therapy was stopped. Later, in a prospective uncontrolled study, 14 patients experiencing an HCV-related GN were treated with IFN-α for 6–12 months [26]. Overall, proteinuria significantly decreased, while renal function remained stable. In 11 patients, sera were tested for HCV RNA while on this therapy. Patients who became cleared of HCV RNA (n = 6) had a better outcome compared to those who remained HCV RNA positive (n = 5). However, virological and renal relapses were observed after completing the therapy. In this study, in 5 patients, the use of oral prednisone, in addition to IFN-α, had no effect on renal function. In contrast, steroid pulses had a beneficial effect in 2 patients. Finally, the use of cytotoxic agents, with or without plasma exchange, was associated with a high rate of death and a flare-up in HCV viremia [26].

Interferon-α and Ribavirin

During the last few years, a combined therapy of IFN-α, especially peg-α-IFN, with ribavirin, has become the gold standard of HCV treatment because it has been found to be more effective than IFN-α alone. This has prompted physicians to treat HCV-related GN with this combination. However, published case reports and uncontrolled studies have only included small numbers of patients so far.

In a prospective uncontrolled study, 20 patients presenting with MPGN (n = 17), MGN (n = 2), and mesangioproliferative GN (n = 1) were treated with

IFN-α and either with or without ribavirin [27]. All patients were given IFN-α 3 MU three times weekly. In cases of persistent HCV RNA at 3 months, ribavirin was added at the daily dose of 15 mg/kg; treatment was continued for 12 months. Four out of the 20 patients became HCV RNA negative within the first 3 months and, consequently, did not receive ribavirin therapy. Only one out of the 16 remaining patients who additionally received ribavirin became cleared of HCV RNA within the serum. Seven patients underwent a ribavirin dose reduction due to adverse events, mainly hemolytic anemia. Overall, both HCV RNA concentration and proteinuria decreased significantly. Serum albumin level, as well as both C3 and C4 complement-component levels, increased significantly. Renal function remained stable. In this study, no data are provided regarding the outcome of renal disease after cessation of anti-HCV therapy.

In order to reduce ribavirin-induced hemolytic anemia, some authors have developed a high-performance liquid chromatography method to monitor the plasma ribavirin level, and have reported on their first treatment with concentration-controlled ribavirin plus IFN-α therapy in HCV-related glomerular disease [28]. The intended trough ribavirin plasma concentration was 10–15 mmol/l. Four patients received standard IFN-α, 2 received peg-α-IFN and ribavirin, and one patient received ribavirin monotherapy because of poor tolerance to IFN-α. Five of the patients had a sustained virological response 6–32 months after antiviral therapy was stopped. One patient relapsed 3 months after completing therapy, whereas one patient who was receiving ribavirin monotherapy did not have a virological response. Serum albumin level normalized in all patients, and proteinuria decreased in all patients. Glomerular filtration rate improved in 3 patients and remained stable in 4 other patients. Despite monitoring ribavirin plasma concentration, the main side effect observed was ribavirin-induced hemolytic anemia, which required a ribavirin dose reduction, low-dose iron, and systematic erythropoietin support. An improvement in renal histology has been also reported in a small number of patients [29].

More recently, 18 patients who had HCV-related cryoglobulinemic MPGN were treated with a combined therapy of standard or peg-α-IFN and ribavirin [30]. After a symptomatic treatment of nephrotic-range proteinuria by furosemide, with or without ACEIs, and with or without plasma exchange that was or was not associated with steroids, 18 patients received anti-HCV therapy, while 7 other patients did not receive any antiviral therapy. Fourteen out of the 18 were treated with standard IFN-α at 3 MU, three times weekly, plus ribavirin at 600–1,000 mg/day, and the 4 other patients received peg-IFN at 1.5 μg/kg weekly with the same dose of ribavirin. The mean duration of anti-HCV therapy was 18 ± 10 months (range 6–24 months). The mean duration of follow-up after completing anti-HCV treatment was 16.7 ± 17.7 months (range 6–30 months). A sustained virological response was observed in 67% of patients. In those patients treated with peg-α-IFN there were three virological responders and one non-responder. After anti-HCV treatment, proteinuria and cryoglobulin levels decreased. In addition, serum albumin level increased significantly in virological responders compared to both nonresponders, who were receiving the combination therapy, and control patients, who were not receiving antiviral treatment. In contrast, serum-creatinine level remained stable in all the groups. These data suggest that antiviral therapy should be given for a long period.

The major side effects of α-IFN can be flu-like symptoms, malaise, myalgia, asthenia, loss of weight, cardiovascular disorders, hematological abnormalities, or neurological disorders. The side effects of α-IFN are enhanced in patients with impaired renal function compared to those with normal renal function. This might be related to differences in α-IFN pharmacokinetics. To date, two molecularly different peg-IFNs are available, i.e. peg-α2a-IFN (Pegasys, Hoffmann-La Roche, Basel, Switzerland) and peg-α2b-IFN (Peg-Intron, Schering-Plough, Berlin Germany). The pegylation of α-IFN results in an increase in its half-life. For both peg-IFN formulations, renal clearance accounts for a relatively smaller proportion of its total clearance compared with non-pegylated IFNs, i.e. 30%. However, peg-α-IFN should be used with caution.

Ribavirin Monotherapy

Despite the absence of a complete and sustained virological response, ribavirin (RBV) monotherapy has been shown to have a beneficial effect on HCV-related glomerulopathy in immunocompetent patients, as well as in renal and liver transplant patients [31].

Ribavirin, when given alone or in association with α-IFN, is responsible for hemolytic anemia, especially in cases of renal function impairment. Thus, it is widely admitted that ribavirin dosage should be adapted to creatinine clearance rather than to body weight, as has been previously recommended. Ribavirin plasma concentration predicts ribavirin-induced anemia. Hence, in patients with impaired renal function, ribavirin should be given with caution. The accumulation of ribavirin induces hemolytic anemia. Severe chronic hemolysis is responsible for iron overload, liver iron deposition, and acceleration in liver fibrosis progression.

Immunosuppressive Therapy

In the past, patients with MC, with or without renal involvement, were treated by plasma exchange to remove circulating cryoglobulins from the plasma and, consequently, to diminish the deposition of immune complexes in the kidney. Cyclophosphamide was also used to improve renal disease by suppressing B lymphocyte stimulation and cryoglobulin production. Steroid pulses were administrated to treat glomerular lesions. Low doses of oral steroids were also given to some patients. Previous uncontrolled studies that included a small number of patients treated with these therapies showed that this regime often controlled the acute phase of the disease, but was often poorly tolerated. The flare-up of HCV RNA concentration observed during immunosuppressive therapy may be harmful to HCV-related liver disease.

Rituximab

Recently, rituximab (RTX), a human-mouse chimeric monoclonal antibody that reacts with the CD20 antigen and, thus, directly and selectively targets the B cells, has proved effective and very well tolerated in patients with B-cell non-Hodgkin lymphomas. Hence, it is used to treat MC and HCV-related cryoglobulinemic MPGN.

Two patients with HCV-related cryoglobulinemic MPGN were treated with RTX at four weekly doses of 375 mg/m^2 [32]. They were unresponsive to conventional treatments, including IFN-α, plasmapheresis, steroids, and either cyclophosphamide or 2-chlorodeoxyadenosine. A rapid response and the disappearance of proteinuria and inactive urinary sediment were observed in one patient who had a recent onset of nephritis. No improvement was noticed in the second patient when RTX was interrupted after two infusions due to a thrombosis of the retinal artery. In the patient who completed RTX therapy, HCV RNA concentration showed minimal fluctuations [32].

Later, 6 patients who had HCV-related cryoglobulinemic GN were treated with RTX [33]. One patient received the standard four weekly doses, and the 5 other patients were treated by the standard protocol, plus two additional infusions at 1 and 2 months later. Proteinuria was decreased in all patients. Serum creatinine level decreased in 2, increased in one, and remained stable in 3 patients. Interestingly, HCV viral load decreased or remained stable in all patients. RTX has been also found to be effective for the treatment of HCV-related type II cryoglobulinemic MPGN when used as a first-line therapy [34].

RTX was efficient in treating de novo cryoglobulinemic MPGN in HCV-positive or -negative renal transplant patients, but is associated with a high rate of infectious complications, which might be related to the impairment of T- and B-cell functions that these patients experience [35]. Further controlled randomized studies are required to define the exact indications of RTX, the dose of RTX required, as well as its long-term effect on HCV-related liver disease.

Acute Severe Disease

During the acute phase, plasmapheresis and steroid pulses might be used to remove circulating cryoglobulins from the plasma and to treat the glomerular infiltration abnormalities, respectively. Even in the absence of controlled randomized studies that compared the use of anti-CD20 monoclonal antibodies, i.e. RTX to IV cyclosphosphamide, RTX therapy should be preferred to cyclophosphamide. This is supported by two very recent publications. In the first, Saadoun et al. [36] examined whether treatment of HCV-related MC may target either the viral trigger (HCV) or the downstream B-cell clonal expansion. In a prospective cohort study, they included 38 HCV-MC patients who received (a) a combination of RTX (375 mg/m^2) once a week for 1 month followed by peg-α-IFN (-2a, 180 μg, or -2b, 1.5 μg/kg) weekly plus RBV (600–1,200 mg) daily for 48 weeks, or (b) peg-α-IFN/ribavirin with the same modalities (n = 55). In the whole population of HCV-MC patients (n = 93), a complete clinical response was achieved in 73.1% (68 of 93), cryoglobulin clearance in 52.7% (49 of 93), and a sustained virological response in 59.1% (55 of 93). Compared with peg-α-IFN/ribavirin, RTX plus peg-α-IFN/ribavirin-treated patients had a shorter time to clinical remission (5.4 ± 4 vs. 8.4 ± 4.7 months, $p = 0.004$), better renal response rates (80.9 vs. 40% of complete response, $p = 0.040$), and higher rates of cryoglobulin clearance (68.4 vs. 43.6%, $p = 0.001$) and clonal VH1–69+ B-cell suppression ($p < 0.01$). Treatment was well tolerated, with 11% of discontinuation resulting from antiviral therapy and no worsening of HCV RNA under RTX. The second study included fewer patients, i.e. 37 who presented with HCV-related MC [37]. The patients were given a combination of peg-α-IFN (-2a: 180 μg or 2b: 1.5 μg/kg) weekly plus RBV (1,000 or 1,200 mg) daily for 48 weeks, with (n = 22) or without (n = 15) RTX (375 mg/m^2) once a week for 1 month followed by two 5 monthly infusions (PIRR). Complete response was achieved in 54.5% (12/22) and in 33.3% (5/15) of patients who received PIRR and peg-α-IFN/RBV, respectively ($p < 0.05$). Clearance of HCV RNA and conversion of B-cell populations from oligoclonal to polyclonal in the liver, bone marrow, and peripheral blood were maintained for up to 3 years in 10 of 12 (83.3%) and in 2 of 5 (40%) patients receiving PIRR and peg-α-IFN/RBV, respectively ($p < 0.01$). Cryoproteins persisted in 22.7% (5/22) of patients with PIRR and in 33.3% (5/15) with peg-α-IFN/RBV despite sustained HCV RNA clearance. No response occurred in the remaining 5 patients of both groups. PIRR therapy is well tolerated and more effective than peg-α-IFN/RBV combination in HCV-related MC. Its effect may last for more than 3 years. The findings of these two studies indicate that RTX combined with peg-α-IFN/ribavirin is well tolerated, is more effective than peg-α-IFN/ribavirin, and has long-lasting effects on HCV-MC.

Recommendations

All patients should be treated with ACEIs in association or not with ARBs, as well as with anti-HCV therapy (table 1). The latter relies on a combined antiviral therapy of standard or peg-α-IFN and ribavirin. We recommend treating patients for at least 48 weeks, and continuing antiviral therapy, even in the absence of a decrease in HCV RNA concentration of 2-log at week 12. Clinicians should be aware that after HCV RNA clearance, cryoglobulinemia may persist for a long period. Ribavirin doses should be adapted according to creatinine clearance in order to avoid its main side effect – hemolytic anemia. Combined antiviral and immunosuppressive therapies may be the treatment of choice for

Table 1. Treatment of HCV-related GN

Patients with moderate proteinuria and non-rapid but progressive renal failure: Symptomatic treatment Anti-HCV therapy for at least 12 months: • Standard α-IFN 3 MU three times/week or peg-IFN-α 1.5 μg/kg/week • Ribavirin: dose adapted to the creatinine clearance or to a trough plasma concentration of 10–15 mmol/l with or without erythropoietin support
Patients with nephrotic range proteinuria and/or progressive renal failure: Symptomatic therapy: furosemide, ACEIs alone or combined with ARBs Plasma exchange: 3 l of plasma three times/week for 2 or 3 weeks RTX: 375 mg/m^2/week for 4 weeks[1] or cyclophosphamide: 2 mg/kg/day for 2–4 months Methylprednisolone pulses: 0.5–1 g/day for 3 consecutive days Anti-HCV therapy (see above)

[1] Additional infusions of RTX might be given in cases of early relapse after conventional therapy.

patients with severe renal disease, i.e. nephrotic syndrome and/or progressive renal failure, or conditions that are refractory to anti-HCV therapy alone.

References

1 Lauer GM, Walker BD: Hepatitis C virus infection. N Engl J Med 2001;345:41–52.
2 Morales JM, Morales E, Andres A, Praga M: Glomerulonephritis associated with hepatitis C virus infection. Curr Opin Nephrol Hypertens 1999;8:205–211.
3 KDIGO Clinical Practice Guidelines for the Prevention, Diagnosis, Evaluation and Treatment of Hepatitis C in Chronic Kidney Disease. Kidney Int 2008;73(suppl 109):S69–S77.
4 Kamar N, Rostaing L, Alric L: Treatment of hepatitis C-virus related glomerulonephritis. Kidney Int 2006;69:436–439.
5 Fabrizi F, Pozzi C, Farina M, et al: Hepatitis C-virus-related glomerulonephritis. Nephrol Dial Transplant 1998;13:1991–1997.
6 El-Serag HB, Hampel H, Yeh C, et al: Extrahepatic manifestations of hepatitis C among United States male veterans. Hepatology 2002;36:1439–1445.
7 Gopalani A, Ahuja TS: Prevalence of glomerulopathies in autopsies of patients infected with the hepatitis C virus. Am J Med Sci 2001;322:57–60.
8 Butt AA, Wang X, Fried LF: HCV infection and the incidence of CKD. Am J Kidney Dis 2011;57:396–402.
9 Satapathy SK, Lingisetty CS, Willimas S: Higher prevalence of chronic kidney disease and shorter renal survival in patients with chronic hepatitis C virus infection. Hepatol Int 2011, Epub ahead of print.
10 Tsui JL, Vittinghoff E, Shlipak MG, et al: Relationship between hepatitis C and chronic kidney disease: results from the Third National Health and Nutrition Examination Survey. J Am Soc Nephrol 2006;17:1168–1174.
11 Huang JF, Chuang WL, Dai CY, et al: Viral hepatitis and proteinuria in an area endemic for hepatitis C and B infections: another chain of link? J Intern Med 2006;260:255–262.

12 Li Cavoli G, Ferrantelli A, Bono L, et al: Incidence of hepatitis C virus infection in patients with chronic kidney disease conservative therapy. Int J Infect Dis 2011;15:e514–e516.

13 Kristiansen MG, Gutteberg TJ, Mortensen, et al: Clinical outcomes in a prospective study of community-acquired hepatitis C virus infection in Northern Norway. Scand J Gastroenterol 2010;45:746–751.

14 D'Amico G: Renal involvement in hepatitis C infection: cryoglobulinemic glomerulonephritis. Kidney Int 1998;54:650–671.

15 Cacoub P, Costedoat-Chalumeau N, Lidove O, et al: Cryoglobulinemia vasculitis. Curr Opin Rheumatol 2002;14:29–35.

16 Davda R, Peterson J, Weiner R, et al: Membranous glomerulonephritis in association with hepatitis C virus infection. Am J Kidney Dis 1993;22:452–455.

17 Perico N, Cattaneo D, Bikbov B, Remuzzi G: Hepatitis C infection and chronic renal diseases. Clin J Am Soc Nephrol 2009;4:207–220.

18 Cao Y, Zhang Y, Wang S, Zou W: Detection of the hepatitis C virus antigen in kidney tissue from infected patients with various glomerulonephritis. Nephrol Dial Transplant 2009;24:2745–2751.

19 Hoch B, Jukneviciuos I, Liapis H: Glomerular injury associated with hepatitis C infection: a correlation with blood and tissue HCV-PCR. Semin Diagn Pathol 2002;19:175–187.

20 Sansonno D, Lauletta G, Montrone M, et al: Hepatitis C virus RNA and core protein in kidney glomerular and tubular structures isolated with laser capture microdissection. Clin Exp Immunol 2005;140:498–506.

21 Wornle M, Schmid H, Banas B, et al: Novel role of toll-like receptor 3 in hepatitis C-associated glomerulonephritis. Am J Pathol 2006;168:370–385.

22 Abou-Zeid AA, El-Sayegh HK: Toll-like receptor 3 gene expression in Egyptian patients with glomerulonephritis and hepatitis C virus infection. Scand J Clin Lab Invest 2011;71:456–461.

23 Merkle M, Ribeiro A, Wornle M: TLR3-dependent regulation of cytokines in human mesangial cells: a novel role for IP-10 and TNF-(alpha) in hepatitis C-associated glomerulonephritis. Am J Physiol Renal Physiol 2011;301:F57–F69.

24 Ghany MG, Strader DB, Thomas DL, Seef LB: AASLD practice guidelines. Diagnosis, management, and treatment of hepatitis C: an update. Hepatology 2009;49:1335–1374.

25 Misiani R, Bellavita P, Fenili D, et al: Interferon alfa-2a therapy in cryoglobulinemia associated with hepatitis C virus. N Engl J Med 1994;330:751.

26 Johnson, RJ, Gretch, DR, Couser, WG, et al: Hepatitis C virus-associated glomerulonephritis. Effect of alpha-interferon therapy. Kidney Int 1994;46:1700.

27 Sabry AA, Sobh, MA, Sheaashaa HA, et al: Effect of combination therapy (ribavirin and interferon) in HCV-related glomerulopathy. Nephrol Dial Transplant 2002;17:1924.

28 Bruchfeld A, Lindahl K, Stahle L, et al: Interferon and ribavirin treatment in patients with hepatitis C-associated renal disease and renal insufficiency. Nephrol Dial Transplant 2003;18:1573.

29 Rossi P, Bertani T, Baio P, et al: Hepatitis C virus-related cryoglobulinemic glomerulonephritis: long-term remission after antiviral therapy. Kidney Int 2003;63:2236.

30 Alric L, Plaisier E, Thebault S, et al: Influence of antiviral therapy in hepatitis C virus-associated cryoglobulinemic MPGN. Am J Kidney Dis 2004;43:617.

31 Pham HP, Feray C, Samuel D, et al: Effects of ribavirin on hepatitis C-associated nephrotic syndrome in four liver transplant recipients. Kidney Int 1998;54:1311.

32 Zaja F, De Vita S, Mazzaro C, et al: Efficacy and safety of rituximab in type II mixed cryoglobulinemia. Blood 2003;101:3827.

33 Roccatello D, Baldovino S, Rossi D, et al: Long-term effects of anti-CD20 monoclonal antibody treatment of cryoglobulinaemic glomerulonephritis. Nephrol Dial Transplant 2004;19:3054.

34 Quartuccio L, Soardo G, Romano G, et al: Rituximab treatment for glomerulonephritis in HCV-associated mixed cryoglobulinaemia: efficacy and safety in the absence of steroids. Rheumatology (Oxford) 2006;45:842.
35 Basse, G, Ribes, D, Kamar, N, et al: Rituximab therapy for de novo mixed cryoglobulinemia in renal-transplant patients. Transplantation 2005;80:1560.
36 Saadoun D, Resche Rigon M, Sene D, et al: Rituximab plus Peg-interferon-alpha/ribavirin compared with Peg-interferon-alpha/ribavirin in hepatitis C-related mixed cryoglobulinemia. Blood 2010;116:326–334.
37 Dammacco F, Tucci FA, Lauletta G, et al: Pegylated interferon-alpha, ribavirin, and rituximab combined therapy of hepatitis C virus-related mixed cryoglobulinemia: a long-term study. Blood 2010;116:343–353.

Prof. Lionel Rostaing
Department of Nephrology, Dialysis, and Organ Transplantation Unit, CHU Rangueil
Toulouse University Hospital
1 Avenue Jean Poulhès, TSA 50032
FR–31059 Toulouse Cedex 9 (France)
Tel. +33 5 61 32 25 84, E-Mail rostaing.l@chu-toulouse.fr

Morales JM (ed): Hepatitis C in Renal Disease, Hemodialysis and Transplantation.
Contrib Nephrol. Basel, Karger, 2012, vol 176, pp 24–34

Hepatitis C-Induced Renal Disease in Patients with AIDS: An Emergent Problem

Manuel Praga · Elena Gutiérrez Solís · Enrique Morales

Nephrology Division, Hospital Universitario 12 de Octubre, Instituto de Investigación Hospital 12 de Octubre, Universidad Complutense de Madrid, Madrid, Spain

Abstract

Cryoglobulinemic membranoproliferative glomerulonephritis (MPGN) is the more characteristic renal disease associated with hepatitis C virus (HCV) infection. Patients infected with human immunodeficiency virus (HIV) can present, in addition to HIV-associated nephropathy, different types of immune complex glomerulonephritis, including MPGN, IgA nephropathy, non-collapsing focal segmental glomerulosclerosis, membranous nephropathy and lupus-like glomerulonephritis. On the other hand, the incidence of hypertensive nephrosclerosis, diabetic nephropathy and decreased renal function similar to that of elderly patients is increasingly recognized among HIV-infected patients. In spite of the fact that HCV coinfection in HIV patients is a very common problem, affecting approximately 30% of HIV-infected patients, information about the role of HCV in renal diseases of HIV-infected patients is scant. A large proportion of HIV patients with glomerular diseases are coinfected with HCV, and the latter is likely the responsible agent in those cases of cryoglobulinemic MPGN reported in HIV-infected patients. Participation of HCV in other types of HIV-related glomerular diseases is uncertain. Patient and renal survival in glomerular diseases of patients coinfected with HIV and HCV is very poor, but some studies suggest that antiretroviral therapy might change this dismal prognosis. Information about the effect of specific anti-VHC therapy or immunosuppressive agents in these patients is very limited.

Introduction

Both hepatitis C virus (HCV) and human immunodeficiency virus (HIV) infections can induce different types of renal complications. The main clinical characteristics of renal diseases associated with either of these infections, as well as the results of different treatments in every condition have been the subject of a considerable number of studies. However, literature about renal complications in patients coinfected with both HCV and HIV is comparatively very scarce. This is surprising, because coinfection with HCV in HIV patients is a very common problem: it has been estimated that approximately 30% of HIV-infected patients are also coinfected with HCV [1]. The fact that both viruses share the same routes of transmission explains the high prevalence of coinfection. On the other hand, the prevalence of HCV coinfection is very variable among HIV-positive patients, ranging from less than 10% to higher than 70%. Patient risk profile largely explains these wide variations: HIV-infected patients who are addicts to illicit intravenous drugs and those practicing unsafe and promiscuous sex exhibit the higher ranges of HCV coinfection, whereas those patients in whom HIV was acquired through other routes have a comparatively lower rates of coinfection. The route of transmission also has an important role in the sequence of infections: intravenous drug users typically acquire HCV before HIV, whereas HIV commonly precedes HCV in men who have sex with men [2].

Coinfection with HCV and HIV has a number of important consequences on the prognosis and management of affected patients. First, infection with HIV accelerates the progression of HCV-induced liver disease, mainly through an increased fibrosis. Several studies have shown that morbidity and mortality due to HCV-induced liver disease are significantly higher among patients with concomitant infection with HIV [3]. The immunosuppressive effect of HIV infection as well as the increased synthesis of pro inflammatory cytokines are the main pathogenic mechanisms that explain this accelerated course to end-stage liver failure. Some data suggest that hepatocellular carcinoma appears at a younger age and has a worse prognosis in HCV/HIV coinfected patients than in those with HCV infection alone. On the other hand, antiretroviral therapy has a beneficial effect on the progression of liver disease [4], although the presence of HCV-related chronic liver disease could enhance the hepatotoxicity of some antiretroviral agents.

Conversely, some studies have suggested a detrimental influence of HCV infection on the progression to a new AIDS-defining illness or death in HIV patients [5], although other studies have not reproduced these findings [6]. It is possible that the HCV viral load could explain these differences because a clear correlation has been found between HCV viral load and the risk of progression to AIDS and death in HIV-infected patients [7].

Renal Disease in HIV-Infected Patients

HIV-Associated Nephropathy

A collapsing form of focal glomerulosclerosis, the so called HIV-associated nephropathy (HIVAN), has been considered the most frequent and most representative glomerular disease in HIV-infected patients [8, 9]. Black patients infected with HIV are much more prone to the development of HIVAN than patients from other ethnicities. Typically, HIVAN presents as a nephrotic syndrome that, in the absence of treatment, is accompanied by a rapid worsening of renal function. Renal biopsies show a collapsing focal glomerulosclerosis, with striking podocyte hypertrophy and tubulointerstitial changes [10]. Isolated deposits of IgM and C3 are observed on immunofluorescence, and no immune complex deposits are found on electron microscopy studies. Although formerly considered as a pathognomonic manifestation of HIVAN, collapsing focal glomerulosclerosis with similar histological changes has been reported as a complication of other viral infections, cancers, drugs and systemic diseases.

Cumulating evidence suggests that HIV infection by itself is responsible for HIVAN. HIV-related antigens have been identified in glomerular cells of patients with HIVAN and in transgenic animal models of HIVAN; expression of HIV genes is sufficient to promote glomerulosclerosis. However, genetic predisposition (particularly among black patients) appears to be crucial for the development of HIVAN after HIV infection.

Antiretroviral therapy has remarkably improved the dismal prognosis of HIVAN that first series of patients reported [11, 12]. Although no prospective, controlled studies have been performed, several cohort studies strongly suggest that this therapy slows the progression of renal impairment and might even prevent the occurrence of HIVAN. In addition, blockade of the renin-angiotensin system has proven to be effective in these patients, by decreasing proteinuria and slowing the progression of renal failure [13].

Glomerular Diseases Other Than HIVAN

After the initial descriptions of HIVAN, several clinical reports alerted about an increased incidence of different types of immune complex glomerulonephritis (GN) in HIV-infected patients [14]. Unlike HIVAN, these GN have no racial predisposition. Clinical presentation and analytical findings, as summarized in table 1, can orientate towards a particular type of GN, but in most of the cases a renal biopsy is indicated to establish the precise diagnosis and to provide important data for prognosis and treatment in every particular case. Series of HIV-infected patients with biopsy-proven IgA nephropathy (IgAN), membranous nephropathy (MN), non-collapsing forms of focal segmental glomerulosclerosis (FSGS), postinfectious GN and membranoproliferative GN (MPGN) have been reported [14–19]. Although their precise incidence cannot be established, it is likely that most of them, if not all, have an increased prevalence among HIV-infected patients in comparison with normal, non-HIV-infected population. There are several factors that could explain this greater predisposition: on one hand, coinfection with other viruses, particularly VHC and VHB, has been found in a large proportion of HIV patients presenting immune complex GN. In some types of GN, like MPGN, these viral infections different from HIV have a

Table 1. Summary of the most important clinical and analytical findings in glomerular diseases of HIV-infected patients

	MPGN	IgAN	FSGS	MN	APGN	Lupus like	HIVAN
Nephrotic syndrome	+++	–	+++	++++	+	++++	++++
Macroscopic hematuria	++	++++	–	–	+++	++	–
AUA	++	++	+	+	–	+	+
ARF	+	++	+	+	+++	+	+
HT/MHT	+	+++	+	+	+	+	+
Hypo-complementemia	+++	–	–	–	++++	+	–
Cryoglobulins+	+++	–	–	–	+	+	–
HCV/HBV coinfection	++++	+	+	++	–	++	–

MPGN = Membranoproliferative GN; IgAN = IgA nephropathy; FSGS = focal segmental glomerulosclerosis; MN = membranous GN; APGN = acute postinfectious GN; HIVAN = HIV nephropathy; AUA = asymptomatic urinary abnormalities; ARF = acute renal failure; HT = hypertension; MHT = malignant hypertension. The number of crosses indicates the incidence/severity of every symptom or finding.

predominant etiologic role: this has been clearly demonstrated in VHC-related cryoglobulinemic MPGN [20]. In contrast, the pathogenic role of VHC and VHB in other types of GN is less clear. The increased incidence of acute infectious processes among HIV patients explains why these patients are more prone to the occurrence of acute postinfectious GN. On the other hand, some specific immunologic disturbances induced by HIV infection might be the responsible factor for other types of GN. Thus, IgA antibodies against some HIV antigens could be implicated in the pathogenesis of HIV-related types of IgAN, and specific HIV antigens and their specific IgA antibodies have been demonstrated in the mesangial deposits of some patients [16].

The particular predisposition of HIV-infected patients to the development of immune complex GN is well illustrated by those patients, most of them presenting with aggressive clinical manifestations (nephrotic syndrome, macroscopic hematuria, acute renal failure) in whom renal biopsy shows a massive deposit of immune complexes along the glomerular capillary walls accompanied by a remarkable hypercellularity of endothelial and mesangial origin. Immunofluorescence and electron microscopy confirm the massive presence of immune complexes. Since the histologic picture could not be included in the different types of GN commented above, the term 'lupus-like' GN has been proposed for these patients, in spite the fact that anti-nuclear and anti-DNA antibodies are characteristically negative and that there are no extrarenal manifestations of systemic lupus erythematosus [18]. It has been speculated that infectious antigens could promote the formation and deposition of immune complexes and that HIV infection by itself (through the deposition of some antigens in the glomeruli as 'planted antigens') could unleash the immune response.

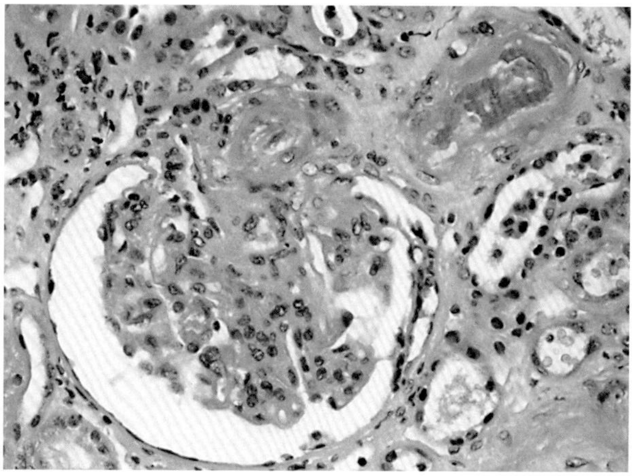

Fig. 1. Mesangioproliferative GN and fibrinoid necrosis of arteriolar walls in a patient coinfected with HIV and HCV who presented with deteriorating renal function and MHT. Immunofluorescence showed predominant deposits of IgA. Final diagnosis, IgAN presenting as MHT. Hematoxylin-eosin stain. ×400.

In general, clinical and analytical findings of immune complex GN in HIV-infected patients are similar to those of primary forms of the disease. However, there are some peculiarities that deserve to be mentioned. One of them is the striking frequency of malignant hypertension (MHT) occurrence (fig. 1). In one study [21], 33% of biopsy-proven GN other than HIVAN in HIV patients presented with MHT (severe hypertension and grade III–IV hypertensive retinopathy). In comparison with HIV-associated GN without MHT, they showed a significantly higher blood pressure at presentation, a higher finding of IgAN and of malignant nephrosclerosis in renal biopsies, a higher viral load and a lower CD4+ cell count at the end of follow-up and a worse patient and renal survival. Although the association of HIV-related IgAN with MHT was particularly striking (approximately 60% of the patients presented with MHT), the occurrence of MHT among other types of GN in HIV patients was also remarkable, ranging from 18 to 25% in patients with MPGN, FSGS and MN [21].

It is possible that HIV infection by itself plays a pathogenic role in this peculiar predisposition to MHT, considering the significantly higher viral load found among the patients who presented with MHT. Another possible pathogenic pathway could rely on the known higher incidence of thrombotic microangiopathy among HIV patients [22]. Both thrombotic microangiopathy and MHT could be interpreted as clinical manifestations of a systemic endothelial injury, due to a direct toxic effect of HIV, other infectious agents (particularly HCV and HBV) or other factors (such as drug addictions) linked to the environment of HIV infection. On the other hand, the presence of antiphospholipid antibodies is common among HIV patients, and these auto-antibodies could play a role in endothelial vascular damage preceding the development of MHT.

Information about treatment of HIV-associated immune complex GN is very scarce. As in most idiopathic types of GN, blockade of the renin-angiotensin-aldosterone system should be fundamental, particularly considering the tendency to the occurrence of MHT. On the other hand, the indication of immunosuppressive regimens, as indicated in some presentations of idiopathic GN, should be tempered in HIV patients given the higher risk of infectious complications. More clinical information is clearly needed.

Non-Glomerular Renal Diseases

Many non-glomerular renal complications have been reported as relatively common among HIV-infected patients: acute kidney injury due to functional factors, drug-induced acute and chronic tubular damage, antiretroviral-induced crystalluria, acute drug-induced interstitial nephritis, interstitial nephropathies caused by infectious agents, tumoral interstitial infiltration or obstructive nephropathy caused by tumors are some of the more important.

Of particular importance is the worrying incidence of diabetic nephropathy and hypertensive nephrosclerosis among HIV patients. In some studies, these entities have been found in approximately 5% of renal biopsies [23]. In addition, the prevalence of microalbuminuria in nondiabetic, normotensive HIV-infected patients appears to be greater than in normal population. Since microalbuminuria is a demonstrated risk factor for the occurrence of cardiovascular events, this finding is of considerable importance. It is thought that metabolic disturbances induced by antiretroviral treatment (insulin resistance, dyslipidemia, changes in body fat distribution) might play an important role in the appearance of diabetes, nephrosclerosis and microalbuminuria. These metabolic disturbances could also be implicated in the common finding of a decreased glomerular filtration rate without significant amounts of proteinuria and with a generally normal urinary sediment among HIV patients. This constellation of renal abnormalities (hypertensive nephrosclerosis, diabetic nephropathy, decreased renal function) resembles the increasingly recognized worldwide occurrence of chronic kidney disease, diabetic and hypertensive nephropathy among elderly. Very interestingly, the same findings have been reported in HIV-infected cohorts of Sub-Saharan Africa not receiving antiretroviral therapy [24], suggesting that HIV infection by itself could induce these metabolic disturbances and their cardiovascular and renal consequences.

Hepatitis C-Induced Renal Disease in HIV-Infected Patients

As explained elsewhere in this book, cryoglobulinemic MPGN is the characteristic glomerular disease associated with HCV infection. The systemic vasculitic manifestations typical of mixed cryoglobulinemia (skin purpura, arthralgias, Raynaud and in more severe cases skin necrosis and even pulmonary hemorrhage) as well as the characteristic analytical findings (hypocomplementemia, increased rheumatoid factor, circulating type II cryoglobulins) are present in many patients [25]. The glomerular involvement shows the typical morphologic appearance of cryoglobulinemic MPGN: mesangial proliferation, double contour images in glomerular capillaries, IgG, IgM and C3 deposits on immunofluorescence, presence of subendothelial electron-dense deposits on electron microscopic examination, cryoglobulin thrombus occluding capillary lumens and occasional vasculitis affecting extraglomerular vessels. Clinical presentation is very variable, ranging from persistent nonnephrotic proteinuria and microhematuria with normal renal function to nephrotic syndrome and macroscopic hematuria accompanied by acute renal failure.

The presence of the above summarized clinical and analytical findings in a patient coinfected with HCV and HIV should lead to the suspicion of an HCV-induced cryoglobulinemic MPGN that will be confirmed in most of the cases by renal biopsy. However, as explained before, HIV-infected patients, independent of whether they are coinfected with HCV or not, can present different types of immune complex GN, with protean morphologic appearances and very variable clinical manifestations. Therefore, glomerular disorders in patients coinfected with HCV and HIV need a careful differential diagnosis and, if not contraindicated, the performance of a renal biopsy.

Aside from typical cryoglobulinemic MPGN, the pathogenic involvement of HCV in other glomerular diseases is more controversial [25]. Some HCV-infected patients present with typical MPGN in the absence of circulating cryoglobulins or other clinical and analytical manifestations of cryoglobulinemia. Fibrillary and immunotactoid glomerulopathies have been linked to the presence of HCV infection in several patients, although a direct pathogenic relationship has not been demonstrated. Finally, although HCV infection has been invoked as a pathogenic contributor in patients with MN and other types of GN, the evidence is very weak or absent, and the presence of HCV could be a mere coincidence.

In spite of the importance of HCV coinfection in HIV patients, the number of clinical studies about renal diseases in patients coinfected with HCV and HIV is regrettably scarce. Morales et al. [26] reported on 3 Caucasian patients with HCV-HIV coinfection who showed an MPGN on renal biopsy. Circulating cryoglobulins were detected in all of them, although systemic manifestations were only present in one. Renal disease was aggressive in 2 patients, with nephrotic syndrome and deteriorating renal function. One of them received corticosteroids later on her clinical course; no improvement was detected and the patient started chronic dialysis. Another patient was treated with methylprednisolone pulses followed by high oral corticosteroid doses immediately after the first renal biopsy. A remarkable improvement of renal function and partial remission of nephrotic syndrome were observed. The third patient (who showed a type III MPGN, with immune deposits on both sides of the glomerular basement membrane) presented with nonnephrotic proteinuria and normal renal function. He was treated with an ACE inhibitor, showing a marked and sustained proteinuria decrease and a long-term stable normal renal function. No patient received specific anti-HCV treatments.

Stokes et al. [27] reported 12 HIV and HCV coinfected intravenous drug users, 7 blacks and 5 Hispanics, who presented with proteinuria, microhematuria, and elevated serum creatinine. Edema, hypertension, and hypocomplementemia were noted in the majority of patients, and 42% of patients had cryoglobulinemia. Ten individuals had evidence of past hepatitis B viral infection, but none had persistent hepatitis B surface antigenemia. Renal biopsy showed MPGN in 5, mesangial proliferative GN in 5, MN in one, and collapsing glomerulopathy with immune complex deposits in one patient. HCV RNA was detected in the renal tissue and/or serum of 9 of the 11 patients tested. Three patients died and 5 patients progressed to end-stage renal failure in the course of follow-up with a mean time to dialysis of 8.4 months after biopsy.

Cheng et al. [28] reported on 14 patients coinfected with HCV and HIV who were referred to their institution because of renal disease. Thirteen out of 14 (93%) were African-Americans, and all of them were intravenous drug users. Mean CD4+ T cells were 238 ± 167/μl and 6 (43%) had AIDS at presentation. Clinical manifestations of renal disease were severe (nephrotic syndrome with renal insufficiency in 10, chronic renal insufficiency in 2, acute renal failure in one and uremia in one) and extrarenal symptoms of systemic cryoglobulinemia were uncommon. Hypocomplementemia was detected in 6 patients and cryoglobulinemia in 4. Renal biopsies showed an MPGN in 11 patients; in 6 of them, it showed the characteristics of a type III MPGN, with immune complexes deposited on both sides of glomerular basement membrane. In the remaining 3 patients, the diagnosis was an MN but accompanied by several atypical findings: lesions of focal glomerulosclerosis with collapsing features, exudative and proliferative changes and mesangial and subendothelial deposits in addition to the typical subepithelial deposits of MN. Alpha-interferon was administered to 3 patients, without clear beneficial effects. No patient received sustained treatment with renin-angiotensin blockers or corticosteroids. The clinical course was characterized by a rapid progression to chronic dialysis or death in a majority of patients. Median time to onset of dialysis or death was 5.8 months. The authors compared this poor survival with that of a historical cohort of patients with HCV infection and renal disease, not infected with HIV, in whom 10-year survival (free of death or chronic renal failure) was 49%.

Gutiérrez et al. [19] reported 27 HIV-infected patients in whom a renal biopsy had been performed because of data suggesting a glomerular disease. The majority of patients were white (88%), young (age 38 ± 5 years), and men (85%). Nineteen (70%) were intravenous drug users. Coinfection with HCV was found in 23 (85%) and with HBV in 10 (37%). Nephrotic syndrome was observed in 52% and deteriorating renal function in 59%. Nine patients presented with MHT (4 of them having IgAN in renal biopsy). The following types of GN were found among those patients coinfected with HIV and HCV: MPGN in 8, IgAN in 6, non-collapsing FSGS in 5, HIVAN in 2 and MN in 2. All the patients with MPGN had coinfection HIV/HCV, but the presence of coinfection was also common in IgAN (100%), FSGS (71%), HIVAN (50%) and MN (100%). Circulating cryoglobulins were detected in 8 patients (6 with MPGN on renal biopsy, 1 with IgAN and 1 with FSGS). No patient received specific therapy for HCV infection. A majority of patients (81%) were treated with renin-angiotensin blockers, and 24 (89%) were receiving antiretroviral therapy for HIV infection at the end of follow-up. In addition, 8 patients (29%) received corticosteroids at initial presentation. Three patients died and 8 progressed to chronic dialysis. In the remaining 16 patients (59%), renal function remained stable during follow-up.

Coinfection with HCV among HIV patients could have implications beyond glomerular diseases. A study performed in 2,684 HIV-infected women showed that 952 (35%) were found to be HCV seropositive. For 180 women with CKD at baseline (eGFR <60 ml/min/1.73 m^2), being HCV seropositive was independently associated with a more rapid decline in renal function [29]. However, coinfection with HCV had no influence on the progression of renal disease in patients with normal renal function.

In summary, the role of HCV coinfection in renal diseases of HIV-infected patients is difficult to ascertain. HIV-infected patients suffer a number of different immune complex glomerular diseases in addition to the classical first-reported HIVAN: MPGN, IgAN, non-collapsing FSGS, MN, or 'lupus-like' GN. Clinical presentation is aggressive in a majority of patients. The pathogenic implication of other viral infections, such as HCV, is not clear, and there is a remarkable scarcity of clinical and investigational information. The majority of patients coinfected with HIV and HCV in whom an MPGN was found in renal biopsy had circulating cryoglobulins and, therefore, these cases could be interpreted as HCV-related cryoglobulinemic MPGN, as in non-HIV-infected patients. However, systemic manifestations of cryoglobulinemia appear to be uncommon, and there is very limited information about the results of specific anti-HCV treatment. On the other hand, HCV could also play a pathogenic role in immune complex glomerular diseases other than MPGN.

Glomerular diseases in patients coinfected with HIV/HCV have shown a dismal prognosis, with a very poor patient and renal survival [26–28]. However, the majority of patients reported in these series did not receive antiretroviral treatment. In the only published series in which a majority of patients were treated with antiretroviral therapy [19], prognosis appeared to be significantly better than in previous reports. Taking into account the positive experience reported in HIVAN and the limited experience in other glomerular diseases, antiretroviral therapy should be prescribed to all HIV patients with glomerular diseases, independent of whether they are or not coinfected with HCV. Regarding specific anti-HCV therapy in HIV-infected patients, several studies and recommendations have been developed, but always focused on HCV-induced liver diseases [30]. Information about the results of anti-HCV therapy in patients coinfected with HIV and suffering glomerular diseases (particularly in those showing MPGN) is urgently needed. While awaiting such information, it appears to be logical to recommend such therapy (interferon, ribavirin) in patients with a biopsy-proven MPGN, circulating cryoglobulins and severe presentations of renal disease (nephrotic syndrome, deteriorating renal function) [25]. Corticosteroids and other immunosuppressive agents, particularly rituximab, have been suggested to induce a beneficial effect in patients with HCV-related cryoglobulinemic MPGN [25], but information about such therapies in patients coinfected with HIV is very limited. In addition, severe side effects may be common in HIV-infected patients receiving immunosuppression.

Acknowledgement

This review was partially supported by grants from Fondo de Investigaciones Sanitarias (FIS 10/02668) and Asociación para la Investigación y Tratamiento de las Enfermedades Renales (AITER).

References

1 Sherman KE, Rouster SD, Chung RT, Rajicic N: Hepatitis C Virus prevalence among patients infected with Human Immunodeficiency Virus: a cross-sectional analysis of the US adult AIDS Clinical Trials Group. Clin Infect Dis 2002;34:831–837.

2 Amon JJ, Garfein RS, Ahdieh-Grant L, et al: Prevalence of hepatitis C virus infection among injection drug users in the United States, 1994–2004. Clin Infect Dis 2008;46:1852–1858.

3 Sulkowski MS, Mehta SH, Torbenson MS, et al: Rapid fibrosis progression among HIV/hepatitis C virus-co-infected adults. AIDS 2007;21:2209.

4 Bräu N, Salvatore M, Ríos-Bedoya CF, et al: Slower fibrosis progression in HIV/HCV-coinfected patients with successful HIV suppression using antiretroviral therapy. J Hepatol 2006;44:47–55.

5 Greub G, Ledergerber B, Battegay M, et al: Clinical progression, survival, and immune recovery during antiretroviral therapy in patients with HIV-1 and hepatitis C virus coinfection: the Swiss HIV Cohort Study. Lancet 2000;356:1800–1805.

6 Sulkowski MS, Moore RD, Mehta SH, et al: Hepatitis C and progression of HIV disease. JAMA 2002;288:199–206.

7 Tedaldi EM, Baker RK, Moorman AC, et al: Influence of coinfection with hepatitis C virus on morbidity and mortality due to human immunodeficiency virus infection in the era of highly active antiretroviral therapy. Clin Infect Dis 2003;36:363–367.

8 D'Agati V, Appel GB: HIV infection and the kidney. J Am Soc Nephrol 1997;8:138–152.

9 Herman ES, Klotman PE: HIV-associated nephropathy: epidemiology, pathogenesis, and treatment. Semin Nephrol 2003;23:200–208.

10 D'Agati V, Appel GB: Renal pathology of human immunodeficiency virus infection. Semin Nephrol 1998;18:406–421.
11 Wali RK, Drachenberg CI, Papadimitriou JC, Keay S, Ramos E: HIV-1-associated nephropathy and response to highly-active antiretroviral therapy. Lancet 1998;352:783–784.
12 Atta MG, Gallant JE, Rahman MH, et al: Antiretroviral therapy in the treatment of HIV-associated nephropathy. Nephrol Dial Transplant 2006;21:2809–2813.
13 Wei A, Burns GC, Williams BA, Mohammed NB, Visintainer P, Sivak SL: Long-term renal survival in HIV-associated nephropathy with angiotensin-converting enzyme inhibition. Kidney Int 2003;64:1462–1471.
14 Nochy D, Glotz D, Dosquet P, et al: Renal disease associated with HIV infection: a multicentric study of 60 patients from Paris hospitals. Nephrol Dial Transplant 1993;8:11–19.
15 Beaufils H, Jouanneau C, Katlama C, Sazdovith V, Hauw JJ: HIV-associated IgA nephropathy – a postmorten study. Nephrol Dial Transplant 1995;10:35–38.
16 Kimmel PL, Phillips TM, Ferreira-Centeno A, Farkas-Szallasi T, Abraham AA, Garret CT: Idiotypic IgA nephropathy in patients with human immunodeficiency virus infection. N Engl J Med 1992;327:729–730.
17 Enríquez R, Cabezuelo JB, Escolano C, et al: Postinfectious diffuse proliferative glomerulonephritis and acute renal failure in an HIV patient. Clin Nephrol 2004;61:278–281.
18 Haas M, Kaul S, Eustace JA: HIV-associated immune complex glomerulonephritis with 'lupus-like' features: a clinicopathologic study of 14 cases. Kidney Int 2005;67:1381–1390.
19 Gutierrez E, Morales E, Gutierrez ME, et al: Glomerulopathies associated to HIV infection: a Spanish perspective. Nefrologia 2007;27:439–447.
20 Kamar N, Rostaing L, Alric L: Treatment of hepatitis C-virus-related glomerulonephritis. Kidney Int 2006;69:436–439.
21 Morales E, Gutiérrez-Solís E, Gutiérrez E, González R, Martínez MA, Praga M: Malignant hypertension in HIV-associated glomerulonephritis. Nephrol Dial Transplant 2008;23:3901–3907.
22 Alpers CE: Light at the end of the TUNEL: HIV-associated thrombotic microangiopathy. Kidney Int 2003;63:385–396.
23 Szczech LA, Gupta SK, Habash R, et al: The clinical epidemiology and course of the spectrum of renal diseases associated with HIV infection. Kidney Int 2004;66:1145–1152.
24 Wools-Kaloustian K, Gupta SK, Muloma E, et al: Renal disease in an atiretroviral-naïve HIV-infected outpatient population in Western Kenya. Nephrol Dial Transplant 2007;22:2208–2212.
25 Perico N, Cattaneo D, Bikvov B, Remuzzi G: Hepatitis C infection and chronic renal diseases. Clin J Am Soc Nephrol 2009;4:207–220.
26 Morales E, Alegre R, Herrero JC, Morales JM, Ortuño T, Praga M: Hepatitis-C-virus associated cryoglobulinaemic membranoproliferative glomerulonephritis in patients infected by HIV. Nephrol Dial Transplant 1997;12:1980–1984.
27 Stokes MB, Chawla H, Brody RI, et al: Immune complex glomerulonephritis in patients coinfected with human immunodeficiency virus and hepatitis C virus. Am J Kidney Dis 1997;29:514–525.
28 Cheng JT, Anderson HL, Markowitz GS, Appel GB, Poque VA, D'Agati V: Hepatitis C virus-associated glomerular disease in patients with human immunodeficiency virus coinfection. J Am Soc Nephrol 1999;10:1566–1574.
29 Tsui J, Vittinghoff E, Anastos K, et al: Hepatitis C seropositivity and kidney function decline among women with HIV: data from the Women's Interagency HIV Study. Am J Kidney Dis 2009;54:43–50.
30 Torriani FJ, Rodriguez-Torres M, Rockstroh JK, et al: Peginterferon Alfa-2a plus ribavirin for chronic hepatitis C virus infection in HIV-infected patients. N Engl J Med 2004;351:438–450.

Dr. Manuel Praga
Servicio de Nefrología, Hospital 12 de Octubre
Avda de Córdoba, s/n.
ES–28041 Madrid (Spain)
Tel. +34 9139 08383, E-Mail mpragat@senefro.org

Morales JM (ed): Hepatitis C in Renal Disease, Hemodialysis and Transplantation.
Contrib Nephrol. Basel, Karger, 2012, vol 176, pp 35–41

Hepatitis C in Hemodialysis: Epidemiology and Prevention of Hepatitis C Virus Transmission

Michel Jadoul[a] · Guillermina Barril[b]

[a]Cliniques Universitaires Saint Luc, Department of Nephrology, Université Catholique de Louvain, Brussels, Belgium; [b]Department of Nephrology, Hospital Universitario de la Princesa, Madrid, Spain

Abstract

Hemodialysis (HD) patients were recognized as a high risk group for hepatitis C virus (HCV) infection almost immediately after the identification of HCV in 1989. Both transfusional and nosocomial transmission of HCV were then relatively frequent in HD. The dramatic reduction in transfusional transmission of HCV in the 1990s soon underlined the strongly suspected nosocomial risk. Multiple molecular virology reports eventually demonstrated patient to patient transmission. The reinforcement of hygienic precautions and/or isolation strategies was the main subsequent step taken by most HD units. Both incidence and prevalence of HCV then decreased substantially in most western HD units. Currently, incidence is much lower whereas prevalence is largely influenced by the rate of acquisition of HCV prior to starting HD (be it in the remote past). Still, the risk of occasional nosocomial transmission remains. The actual application of basic hygienic precautions remains the cornerstone of the prevention of HCV nosocomial transmission, as reviewed in the recently published KDIGO guidelines on HCV in CKD.

The epidemiology of hepatitis C virus (HCV) infection in hemodialysis (HD) patients has changed dramatically worldwide since the identification of HCV as the main cause of non-A non-B hepatitis in 1989. The understanding of the routes of HCV transmission in HD also has improved. In this chapter, we review the evolution of the epidemiology of HCV in HD over the last 2 decades, as well as the available strategies to prevent HCV transmission to HD patients.

HCV Epidemiology in HD: The 1990s

As soon as serological tests for HCV became available, HD patients were unsurprisingly recognized as a high risk group. This recognition was in line with previous reports of non-A non-B hepatitis outbreaks in HD patients [1]. This high prevalence was undoubtedly partly related to the (at that time) high risk of posttransfusional hepatitis C together with the regular use of transfusions in HD patients [1]. However, multiple arguments also supported ongoing nosocomial transmission in HD units. Indeed, prevalence of HCV infection was strongly correlated with time on dialysis, independent of transfusional burden in some studies, it was higher in HD than in PD or home HD patients, and prevalence was substantial in some studies in never transfused patients [2]. The prevalence and incidence of HCV infection in HD were almost uniformly high in the early 1990s in western countries [2].

With the rapidly improving sensitivity of screening of blood donors, as well as the widespread availability of erythropoiesis-stimulating agents in the early 1990s, the role of transfusions in the transmission of HCV to HD patients probably dramatically decreased, although studies specifically devoted to this topic in HD are few. The risk of posttransfusion hepatitis C was indeed around 0.5% per blood unit in the 1980s and has been shown to drop to around 0.0001% (i.e. one case of hepatitis C per million blood units) in the USA, with similar dramatic improvements in the viral safety of blood in other western countries [3, 4]. As a result, the HD community has become more and more concerned with the nosocomial transmission of HCV within HD units [5–8]. Early reactions to the strong suspicion of nosocomial transmission of HCV in HD varied between countries and units. Some countries such as Spain whose prevalence was initially >30% adopted an isolation of HCV+ patients either by ward or monitor, together with reinforcement of hygienic precautions [9]. Others, like most units in Belgium, just reinforced hygienic precautions [5]. Arguments against isolation for HCV included the long window between HCV infection and seroconversion, the much lower infectivity of HCV than HBV, the potential need of multiple wards for variably B- and/or C-infected HD patients, and the risk of coinfection by multiple HCV genotypes [10]. On the contrary, supporters of isolation strategies claimed that everything that could be done should be done to prevent HCV nosocomial transmission, especially in units with high recent seroconversion rates [9].

Whatever the adopted strategy, the incidence and prevalence of HCV infection soon decreased in many countries [9, 11, 12]. In the absence of randomized controlled trial or even of control group, these A-B or before–after studies cannot claim causality regarding the observed improvement.

As detailed in the next section, the current evidence strongly supports careful hygienic precautions, whereas isolation strategies did not demonstrate an independent protective effect (albeit a detrimental impact remains unproven, and isolation may have contributed to raise awareness of risk of transmission in some settings).

Routes of Nosocomial HCV Transmission: Lessons from Molecular Virology Papers

Nosocomial transmission has, from the mid-1990s on, been unequivocally demonstrated by multiple studies based on phylogenetic analyses of isolates of HCV harvested from patients on HD in the same unit. Studies identified clusters of closely related isolates of HCV both in individual units with high seroconversion rates and in multicenter studies. Some parts of the HCV genome are indeed highly variable, due to frequent mutations like in other RNA viruses such as influenza or HIV, and thus lend themselves to fingerprinting of each isolate or quasi species using sequencing of nucleic acids [13]. Using such an approach, the probability of nosocomial transmission of HCV isolates from a common source can be calculated. Combined with epidemiological data from the unit where isolates of HCV were harvested, this provides scientific evidence to support nosocomial transmission and derive indirect evidence concerning the routes of nosocomial HCV transmission [13].

The KDIGO group thus performed a systematic review of molecular virology papers that included both newly diagnosed HCV+ HD patients from (an) already infected (source) patient(s) and some epidemiological data. Twenty such studies were identified, with between 1 and 22 newly diagnosed cases of HCV. In none of the 20 studies was the specific transmission route conclusively established. This is not surprising, given that the investigations were performed after the event. All studies however suggested failures in infection control procedures to be the probable cause of the new HCV case(s). In only one study was transmission of HCV by the internal fluid pathway of the dialysis machine considered as possible [reviewed in 13]. In contrast, in 18 out of 20 studies, the authors reported that some or all new HCV cases did not share their dialysis machine with the source patient: either they were dialyzed at the same time or the policy of the units assigned them different machines than HCV-positive ones [13]. Thus, internal HD machine circuit appears to play, if any, at most a small role in the nosocomial transmission of HCV HD patients.

The workgroup did not find evidence for a publication bias. It appears therefore licit to generalize from these admittedly small-sized studies to the HD community at large. Accordingly, the KDIGO workgroup concluded that the use of dedicated dialysis machines for HCV infected patients is not recommended (strength of the recommendation: moderate) [13]. Regarding the alternative strategy of isolating HCV-positive patients not only on separate machines but also in a separate ward, the KDIGO workgroup did not find any randomized controlled trials. Still, 2 large prospective observational studies, the DOPPS [14] and the Italian study [7], concluded after multivariate adjustment for potential confounders including the prevalence of HCV infection within the HD unit, that isolation does not protect against HCV transmission to HD patients. Thus, the workgroup concluded that the isolation of HCV-infected patients is not recommended as an alternative to strict infection control procedures for preventing transmission of bloodborn pathogens (strength of the recommendation: weak) [13].

Optimal Strategy to Prevent Nosocomial HCV Transmission in HD

Virtually every single paper devoted to the topic of HCV in HD agrees on the fact that the implementation of hygienic precautions is of critical importance for the prevention of HCV transmission within HD units. These are detailed in the KDIGO guidelines in 2 tables concerning either general hygienic precautions for hemodialysis, or dialysis machines, respectively [13]. These guidelines are freely available at www.kdigo.org. Briefly, staff should wash their hands with soap or an antiseptic handwash and water before and after any contact with a patient or any equipment at the dialysis station. An antiseptic alcohol gel rub is a good alternative if the hands are not visibly contaminated. Staff should in addition wear disposable gloves when caring for a patient or touching any potentially contaminated surfaces at the dialysis stations. Gloves should always be removed when leaving the dialysis station. Single-use items required in the dialysis process should be disposed of after use on one patient. Nondisposable items should be disinfected or dedicated to a single patient. After each session, all potentially contaminated surfaces at the dialysis station should be cleaned with a low level disinfectant if not visibly contaminated. Visibly contaminated surfaces should be disinfected with a stronger agent [13]. Where dialyser reuse is unavoidable, dialysers of HCV-infected patients can be reused provided there is implementation of and adherence to strict infection control procedures (strength of recommendation: weak). Finally, the KDIGO guidelines include recommendations regarding waste management and recommend integrating regular observational audits of infection control procedures in performance reviews of HD units [13]. Indeed, the broad consensus on the hygienic precautions to be adopted does not guarantee their actual application.

Regarding the dialysis machines, the KDIGO guidelines recommend replacing the transducer protector if the filter becomes wet. If any fluid is visible beyond the filter, the machine should be taken out of service after the session so that the internal filter can be changed and the housing disinfected. Disinfection of the internal pathway of a single pass dialysis machine is not considered mandatory unless a blood leak has occurred, but staff should ensure that sufficient time is available between patients for the external surfaces (of environment and machine) to be disinfected [13].

Will the HCV Disappear from HD Units?

Despite the substantial reduction over the last 2 decades in the incidence and prevalence of HCV in HD patients worldwide [5, 9, 11, 12, 15–18], the HCV will stay for additional decades in HD units. Indeed, as the incidence of HCV infection acquired on HD has decreased, it has become more and more apparent in recent years that a substantial proportion of HCV-positive HD patients have been infected by HCV prior to starting any renal replacement therapy [19–23]. The factors accounting for these may include transfusions before the era of appropriate screening of blood and organ donors for hepatitis C (i.e. before 1992 in western countries), intravenous drug use, remote nosocomial (or at least healthcare-related) HCV transmission decades ago, etc. Finally, it should not be forgotten that HCV is a cause of cryoglobulinemic and/or membranoproliferative glomerulonephritis, progressing not infrequently to ESRD [24].

This changing pattern of HCV epidemiology in HD (from acquisition relatively shortly after starting HD in the 1990s to mostly acquired prior to starting HD in the new millennium) may have implications regarding prognosis and treatment of HCV infection too. Indeed, it is well known that most HCV-related complications develop only after decades. Thus, intuitively, the longer average duration of HCV infection in HD patients in recent years than in the 1990s may increase their risk of cirrhosis and hepatocellular carcinoma. This calls for careful follow-up of the liver disease (and potential complications) in such patients [13].

Current Prevalence of HCV in HD Patients

The prevalence of anti-HCV+ is currently below 10% in most but not all countries; very high (>20%) anti-HCV+ rates are still observed in association with societal crisis, war or poor economic status [25–28]. In that context, sustaining a chronic HD program is already a major challenge, and the training of staff for preventing HD-associated HCV transmission is probably suboptimal. In addition, the remarkable viral safety of blood transfusions in western countries should not be assumed to be universal [29].

Attitude when Facing Seroconversion in a Chronic HD Patient

The incidence of seroconversion for HCV is currently low in most western HD units. Still, outbreaks or isolated cases of HCV nosocomial transmission may occur.

A seroconversion for HCV in an HD patient should trigger several questions.

Firstly, did the patient acquire HCV inside or outside the HD unit? Is he or she an intravenous drug user? Did the patient travel for holidays and undergo HD in a high-risk country [30]? Did he/she receive transfusions in this country [29]? If not, was he/she on HD in the same ward at the same time as one or more HCV+ patient(s)? If the answer is yes, molecular virology, performed by many reference centers worldwide, may demonstrate nosocomial transmission.

Alternatively but less likely, was he dialyzed on the same monitor as an HCV+ patient? Finally, and most importantly, is there evidence (even retrospective) of breaches in hygienic precautions? Such an event indeed calls for bolstering of basic, too often neglected, precautions. Simultaneously, additional new cases of HCV infection should be actively searched, preferably by nucleic acid testing [13].

References

1 Jadoul M, Cornu C, van Ypersele de Strihou C: Non-A, non-B hepatitis in dialysis patients: diagnosis, prevention and treatment; in Andreucci VE, Fine LG (eds): International Yearbook of Nephrology 1992. Berlin, Springer, 1991, pp 253–270.

2 Pereira BJ, Levey AS: Hepatitis C virus infection in dialysis and renal transplantation. Kidney Int 1997;51:981–999.

3 Blajchman MA, Vamvakas EC: The continuing risk of transfusion-transmitted infections. N Engl J Med 2006;355:1303–1305.

4 Nübling M, Heiden M, Chudy M, Kress J, Seitz R, Keller-Stanislawski B, Funk MB: Experience of mandatory nucleic acid test (NAT) screening across all blood organizations in Germany: NAT yield versus breakthrough transmissions. Transfusion 2009;49:1850–1858.

5 Jadoul M, Cornu C, van Ypersele de Strihou C, the UCL Collaborative group: Universal precautions prevent hepatitis C virus transmission: a 54 month follow-up of the Belgian multicenter study. Kidney Int 1998;53:1022–1025.

6 Centers for Disease Control and Prevention. Recommendations for preventing transmission of infections among chronic hemodialysis patients. MMWR 2001;50:RR-5.

7 Petrosillo N, Gilli P, Serraino D, Dentico P, Mele A, Ragni P, Puro V, Casalino C, Ippolito G: Prevalence of infected patients and understaffing have a role in hepatitis C virus transmission in dialysis. Am J Kidney Dis 2001;37:1004–1010.

8 Sypsa V, Psichogiou M, Katsoulidou A, Skoutelis G, Moutafis S, Hadjiconstantinou V, Kakavas J, Kalapothaki V, Boletis J, Hatzakis A: Incidence and patterns of hepatitis C virus seroconversion in a cohort of hemodialysis patients. Am J Kidney Dis 2005;45:334–343.

9 Barril G, Traver JA: Decrease in the hepatitis C virus (HCV) prevalence in hemodialysis patients in Spain: effect of time, initiating HCV prevalence studies and adoption of isolation measures. Antiviral Res 2003;60:129–134.

10 Jadoul M: Should hemodialysis patients with hepatitis C virus antibodies be isolated? Semin Dial 1995;8:1–3.

11 Jadoul M, Poignet JL, Geddes C, Locatelli F, Medin C, Krajewska M, Barril G, Scheuermann E, Sonkodi S, Goubeau P, the HCV collaborative group: The changing epidemiology of hepatitis C virus (HCV) infection in haemodialysis: European multicentre study. Nephrol Dial Transplant 2004;19:904–909.

12 Espinosa M, Martn-Malo A, Ojeda R, Santamara R, Soriano S, Aguera M, Aljama P: Marked reduction in the prevalence of hepatitis C virus infection in hemodialysis patients: causes and consequences. Am J Kidney Dis 2004;43:685–689.

13 KDIGO Clinical Practice Guidelines for the prevention, diagnosis, evaluation and treatment of hepatitis C in chronic kidney disease. Kidney Int 2008;73(suppl 109):S1–S99.

14 Fissell RB, Bragg-Gresham JL, Woods JD, Jadoul M, Gillespie B, Hedderwick SA, Rayner HC, Greenwood RN, Akiba T, Young EW: Patterns of hepatitis C prevalence and seroconversion in hemodialysis units from three continents: the DOPPS. Kidney Int 2004;65:2335–2342.

15 Süleymanlar G, Serdengeçti K, Altiparmak MR, Jager K, Seyahi N, Erek E, Turkish Registry of Nephrology, Dialysis, and Transplantation: Trends in renal replacement therapy in Turkey, 1996–2008. Am J Kidney Dis 2011;57:456–465.

16 Sauné K, Kamar N, Miédougé M, Weclawiak H, Dubois M, Izopet J, Rostaing L: Decreased prevalence and incidence of HCV markers in haemodialysis units: a multicentric French survey. Nephrol Dial Transplant 2010;26:2309–2316.

17 Nakai S, Suzuki K, Masakane I, Wada A, et al: Overview of regular dialysis treatment in Japan (as of 31 December 2008). Ther Apher Dial 2010;14:505–540.

18 Johnson DW, Dent H, Yao Q, Tranaeus A, Huang CC, Han DS, Jha V, Wang T, Kawaguchi Y, Qian J: Frequencies of hepatitis B and C infections among haemodialysis and peritoneal dialysis patients in Asia-Pacific countries: analysis of registry data. Nephrol Dial Transplant 2009;24:1598–1603.

19 Bergman S, Accortt N, Turner A, Glaze J: Hepatitis C infection is acquired pre-ESRD. Am J Kidney Dis 2005;45:684–689.

20 Ilçöl B, Ozener C, Avşar M, Ilçol Y, Lawrence R, Ozer A, Cirakoğlu B, Akoğlu E: Hepatitis C infection in patients with chronic renal failure receiving conservative therapy. Nephrol Dial Transplant 1997;12:626.

21 López-Alcorocho JM, Barril G, Ortiz-Movilla N, Traver JA, Bartolomé J, Sanz P, Selgas R, Carreño V: Prevalence of hepatitis B, hepatitis C, GB virus C/hepatitis G and TT viruses in predialysis and hemodialysis patients. J Med Virol 2001;63:103–107.

22 Lemos LB, Perez RM, Lemos MM, Draibe SA, Silva IS, Silva AE, Ferraz ML: Hepatitis C among predialysis patients: prevalence and characteristics in a large cohort of patients. Nephron Clin Pract 2008;108:c135–c140.

23 Iwasa Y, Otsubo S, Sugi O, Sato K, Asamiya Y, Eguchi A, Iwasaki T, Matsuda N, Kikuchi K, Ikebe N, Miwa N, Kimata N, Uchida K, Uchida S, Nitta K, Akiba T: Patterns in the prevalence of hepatitis C virus infection at the start of hemodialysis in Japan. Clin Exp Nephrol 2008;12:53–57.

24 Kamar N, Rostaing L, Alric L: Treatment of hepatitis C-virus-related glomerulonephritis. Kidney Int 2006;69:436–439.

25 Ali I, Siddique L, Rehman LU, Khan NU, Iqbal A, Munir I, Rashid F, Khan SU, Attache S, Swati ZA, Aslam MS: Prevalence of HCV among the high risk groups in Khyber Pakhtunkhwa. Virol J 2011;8:296.

26 Voiculescu M, Iliescu L, Ionescu C, Micu L, Ismail G, Zilisteanu D, Radasan A, Micu G, Pertache I: A cross-sectional epidemiological study of HBV, HCV, HDV and HEV prevalence in the subcarpathian and south-eastern regions of Romania. J Gastrointestin Liver Dis 2010;19:43–48.

27 El-Ottol AEY, Elmanama AA, Ayesh BM: Prevalence and risk factors of hepatitis B and C viruses among haemodialysis patients in Gaza strip, Palestine. Virol J 2010;7:210.

28 Bin Selm S: Prevalence of hepatitis C virus infection among hemodialysis patients in a single center in Yemen. Saudi J Kidney Dis Transplant 2010;21:1165–1168.

29 Prati D: Transmission of hepatitis C virus by blood transfusions and other medical procedures: a global review. J Hepatol 2006;45:607–616.

30 Bhattacharya S, Price N, Boxall E, Adu D, Lipkin G, Smith S, Osman H: Holiday haemodialysis and imported hepatitis C virus infection: a series of sixteen cases in two large haemodialysis units. J Clin Virol 2009;45:296–299.

Prof. Michel Jadoul
Cliniques Universitaires Saint Luc, Department of Nephrology
Université Catholique de Louvain
B-1200 Brussels (Belgium)
E-Mail Michel.Jadoul@uclouvain.be

Morales JM (ed): Hepatitis C in Renal Disease, Hemodialysis and Transplantation.
Contrib Nephrol. Basel, Karger, 2012, vol 176, pp 42–53

Hepatitis C-Related Liver Disease in Dialysis Patients

Fabrizio Fabrizi[a,b] · Vivek Dixit[b] · Piergiorgio Messa[a] · Paul Martin[b]

[a]Division of Nephrology and Dialysis, Maggiore Hospital, IRCCS Foundation, Milano, Italy;
[b]Division of Hepatology, School of Medicine, University of Miami, Miami, Fla., USA

Abstract

Hepatitis C virus (HCV) remains the most common cause of liver damage in patients with chronic kidney disease including patients on long-term dialysis. The natural history of HCV infection in patients with chronic kidney disease is not fully elucidated despite the adverse effect of HCV infection on survival in patients receiving long-term dialysis. A recent meta-analysis of seven observational studies (11,589 patients on dialysis) reported that the summary estimate for adjusted relative risk (all-cause mortality) with anti-HCV antibody was 1.34 with a 95% confidence interval of 1.13–1.59. As a cause of death, hepatocellular carcinoma and liver cirrhosis were significantly more frequent among anti-HCV-positive than -seronegative dialysis patients; the summary estimate for unadjusted liver-related mortality risk was 5.89 (95% confidence interval 1.93–17.99). Impairment of quality of life due to HCV has also been suggested to explain the diminished survival in this setting. Recent data also suggest an excess risk of cardiovascular disease in HCV-infected dialysis patients. Recent evidence supports the notion that the progression of HCV-related liver disease is probably slower in the dialysis population than in non-uremic patients despite the immune compromise conferred from chronic uremia; numerous mechanisms have been mentioned to explain it. It appears that the hemodialysis procedure per se reduces the HCV viral load, and the mechanisms by which this phenomenon occurs remain largely speculative – the intradialytic production of interferon-α, hepatocyte growth factor, or other cytokines provided with antiviral activities have been implicated. This is an area of intense investigation, and further studies are indicated.

The advent of serologic screening of blood by enzyme-linked immunoassays, routine use of erythropoietin for patients with anemia and chronic kidney disease (CKD), and compliance with infection control procedures to prevent the spread of hepatitis C virus (HCV) within dialysis units have helped to reduce the transmission of HCV infection among patients on maintenance dialysis in developed countries [1]. However, HCV infection continues to be the most frequently recognized cause of liver damage in patients with CKD. The aim of this chapter is to review the recent and available evidence on HCV-related liver disease in patients undergoing long-term dialysis.

HCV-Related Liver Disease in Dialysis: Biochemical and Clinical Manifestation

HCV-related liver disease is mostly asymptomatic in patients on long-term dialysis. Some symptoms which typically occur in non-dialysis patients with HCV (i.e. asthenia, fatigue, and cognitive impairment) are frequently in the dialysis population irrespective their HCV serologic status. HCV infection can be evident at biochemical level, as some enzyme levels (serum transaminase and gamma glutamyl transpeptidase, GGTP) are frequently elevated in HCV-infected patients on long-term dialysis. In a large cohort of patients undergoing long-term dialysis in the US (13,664 patients), after adjustment for several covariates including surrogates of MCS (malnutrition-inflammatory complex syndrome), an independent relationship between anti-HCV seropositive status and serum alkaline phosphatase activity was found, OR, 1.01 (95% confidence interval, CI, 1.0–1.02), $p = 0.001$ [2]. Among HCV-infected patients, higher serum intact parathormone levels have been detected, 422 ± 423 vs. 338 ± 356 pg/ml ($p = 0.0001$), which persisted even among African-American patients [3]. These observations have been linked to 'hepatic osteodystrophy' that has been described in non-dialysis subjects with hepatitis [4]. However, dialysis patients have multiple comorbidities (arterial hypertension, gastrointestinal bleeding, anemia, and failure of the vascular access, among others), and clinicians frequently neglect these biochemical alterations in the everyday clinical practice. Cirrhosis is an infrequent event among dialysis patients in western world as it ranges between 1.5 and 2%, according to some international registries [5].

Natural History of HCV in Dialysis Population

The natural history of HCV in patients on maintenance dialysis remains incompletely appreciated. HCV infection in dialysis patients is usually asymptomatic with an apparently indolent course. Because the natural history of HCV extends over decades rather than years even in patients with normal renal function, adverse consequences of chronic HCV infection may not be obvious in patients followed for shorter periods of time. Patients with CKD have higher morbidity and mortality rates than the general population because their average age is higher and because of their frequent comorbidities. The long-term consequences of HCV infection are therefore difficult to assess in this population.

Factors modifying progression of liver disease in patients with CKD include alcohol abuse and coinfection with HBV, HCV, and HIV. Antiviral therapy of HCV in patients on long-term dialysis and elimination of post-transfusion HCV hepatitis hamper the implementation of observational studies with appropriate follow-up. Posttransfusion HCV hepatitis is, in fact, a form of hepatitis in which the timing of acquisition of the virus is likely to be unequivocal.

Biochemical evaluation of HCV infection in patients with CKD is inaccurate. Serum aminotransferase values are typically lower in dialysis patients than the non-uremic populations. Dialysis patients who are HCV viremic have aminotransferase levels greater than those without, although values are still within the 'normal' range. In a series of 394 chronic hemodialysis (HD) patients, serum aspartate aminotransferase activity in bDNA-positive versus -negative patients was 23.8 (95% CI, 60.8–9.3) vs. 17.1 (95% CI, 50.4–5.8), $p = 0.009$, and serum alanine aminotransferase (ALT) activity, 14.4 (95% CI, 48.9–4.3) vs. 9.8 (95% CI, 37.3–2.5) IU/l, $p = 0.008$. Logistic regression analysis showed an association between HCV viremia and ALT activity ($p = 0.01$) [6].

Serum GGTP levels are greater in dialysis patients with HCV and/or HBV infection compared to non-infected patients, but the increase was rather small (85.1 ± 184 vs. 25.8 ± 24 IU/l, $p = 0.001$) and occurred in a minority of patients (41/184 = 22%). Multivariate analysis established a significant and independent relationship between serum GGTP and positive anti-HCV antibody ($p = 0.001$) in a large population of patients on long-term dialysis in northern Italy ($n = 757$) [7].

Clinicians are frequently reluctant to perform liver biopsy in dialysis patients because of concerns about platelet function in chronic uremia. The recent implementation of guidelines recommending antiviral therapy for HCV infection in patients with CKD makes difficult the conduction of longitudinal clinical trials on the natural history of HCV infection in patients with CKD [1].

HCV: Survival and Hemodialysis

Mortality is an unequivocal end point in the natural history of HCV, but data concerning the relationship between HCV infection and risk for death among HCV-infected patients are not abundant. However, longitudinal studies with an appropriate size and follow-up have found an independent and significant relationship between anti-HCV antibody positivity and reduced patient survival [8–11]. A recent meta-analysis of seven observational studies about the effect of anti-HCV serologic status on survival in dialysis patients demonstrated an independent and significant impact of HCV on mortality among patients receiving long-term dialysis (11,589 patients); the summary estimate for relative risk was 1.34 (95% CI, 1.33–1.86) [12]. In all these studies, hepatocellular carcinoma (HCC) and liver cirrhosis were significantly more frequent causes of death in anti-HCV antibody-positive patients on dialysis than in anti-HCV antibody-negative patients on dialysis. The unadjusted overall estimate for the relative risk of liver-related mortality was 5.89 (95% CI, 1.93–17.99, $p < 0.001$) in anti-HCV antibody-positive patients on dialysis relative to their anti-HCV antibody-negative counterparts [12].

A recent study from Australia and New Zealand (n = 23,046) also reported an independent and significant association between anti-HCV-positive serologic status and all-cause mortality over a 10-year follow-up (HR, 1.25, 95% CI 1.07–1.46, p = 0.004) [13]. Hepatic failure was a more common cause of death in the anti-HCV-positive group (adjusted hazard ratio, aHR, 5.79, 95% CI 1.99–16.83, p = 0.001), but this was still infrequent (rate = 0.34 deaths per 100 patients per year). In the anti-HCV-positive group, one of the 9 deaths due to malignancy was to primary liver cancer compared with 12 of 583 deaths due to malignancy in the anti-HCV-negative group. These authors suggested that the majority of dialysis patients who are infected with HCV may not live long enough to die of long-term complications of HCV-related liver disease (i.e. HCC and cirrhosis).

Another population-based survey has been reported by Johnson et al. [14] in dialysis patients (HD and peritoneal dialysis, PD) from Asia-Pacific countries. Analysis of the Japanese cohort (76,201 patients) showed that the presence of anti-HCV antibody was an independent predictor of all-cause mortality (RR, 1.37; 95% CI, 1.15–1.62, p = 0.003). Similarly, in the cohort from Australia and New Zealand (21,487 patients), all-cause mortality was linked to the presence of anti-HCV at baseline (aHR, 1.29; 95% CI, 1.05–1.58, p = 0.016) and acquisition of anti-HCV antibody during the course of dialysis (aHR, 1.27; 95% CI, 1.05–1.55, p = 0.017) [14]. Unfortunately, no information on liver-related or cardiovascular death risk was provided.

These findings are consistent with accumulating evidence from other sources [15, 16]. The Dialysis Outcomes and Practice Patterns Study on patients undergoing regular dialysis in three continents had reported an independent and significant association between positive anti-HCV antibody and mortality risk (adjusted relative risk, aRR, 1.17; $p < 0.0159$) [16].

HCV: Survival and Peritoneal Dialysis

Evidence on the relationship between HCV and survival among patients on PD is even more limited. Wang et al. [17] retrospectively reviewed 538 PD patients from 1996 to 2005. Of these patients, 75 (13.9%) were anti-HCV positive at the beginning of PD. Cox regression analysis suggested that chronic HCV

Table 1. Impact of HCV on survival in dialysis patients: aRR of all-cause mortality

First author	Patients	aRR	Reference year	Country
B. Pereira	496	1.41	1998	US
C. Stehman-Breen	200	1.97	1998	US
E. Nakayama	1,470	1.57	2000	Japan
M. Espinosa	175	1.62	2001	Spain
K. Kalantar-Zadeh	2,778	1.28	2005	US
A. Di Napoli	6,412	1.29	2006	Italy
S.M. Wang	538	2.19	2008	Taiwan

infection was associated with increased 10-year mortality. The adjusted HR of HCV infection was 2.195 (95% CI, 1.486–3.243, p = 0.001). The incidence of liver cirrhosis-related mortality was higher in patients with HCV infection than in those without; however, it was not statistically significant (p = 0.146). HCV infection was not significantly associated with any specific cause of death. The frequency of the three most frequent causes of death (CVD, infection and cancer) was not significantly different in patients with and without HCV (p = 0.597). Serum levels of albumin (3.1 ± 1 vs. 3.4 ± 0.8 mg/dl), cholesterol (178 ± 44 vs. 198 ± 52 mg/dl), and triglyceride (194 ± 12 vs. 212 ± 17 mg/dl) were lower in anti-HCV-positive patients, suggesting that HCV infection might result in increased mortality due to impaired nutritional status.

HCV: Survival and Cardiovascular Disease

Kalantar-Zadeh et al. [3] were the first investigators to establish a relationship between anti-HCV antibody serologic status and cardiovascular mortality. In a population-based survey (2,778 patients undergoing long-term dialysis at DaVita system), the HR for all-cause mortality and cardiovascular death was 1.28 (95% CI, 1.02–1.62, p = 0.03) and 1.48 (95% CI, 1.05–2.08, p = 0.02), respectively, after adjustment for several case-mix parameters. The link between anti-HCV antibody positivity and cardiovascular death was partially mitigated after adjustment for available surrogates of malnutrition-inflammation syndrome, HR, 1.43 (95% CI, 1.00–2.06, p = 0.05). However, the association between anti-HCV positive serologic status and CVD mortality did persist after adjustment for case-mix and MICS covariates, HR = 1.80 (95% CI, 1.1–2.95, p = 0.02), in the subgroup of dialysis patients younger than 65 years (n = 1,551).

In their subsequent survey (13,664 patients on regular dialysis followed during 3 years), the HR of 3-year all-cause mortality related to HCV antibody positivity was 1.25 (95% CI, 1.12–1.39, $p = 0.001$) [2]. The relative risk of cardiovascular disease mortality associated with HCV infection persisted across almost all group of patients, although it did not reach statistical significance.

Interestingly, Scott et al. [13] in another population-based study reached similar conclusions. The predominant cause of death in their cohort was cardiovascular: also, having taken into account patient characteristics including age and pre-existing cardiovascular disease, a significantly increased risk of cardiovascular death among the anti-HCV positive cohort persisted (HR, 1.34, 95% CI, 1.08–1.67, $p = 0.007$). This study differed from other studies as the authors censored their data at the time of transplant in order to remove the potential for confounding by post-transplant outcomes [12]. However, their observation was valid as follow-up of the dialysis cohort continued through the transplantation period (aHR = 1.27, 95% CI, 1.10–1.48).

Another observation is that HCV-infected dialysis patients have a higher prevalence of hypoalbuminemia when compared to non-HCV-infected counterparts. A survey from the US reported a significant difference in serum levels of albumin in their cohort of patients on long-term dialysis (n = 69,294), 3.68 ± 0.45 vs. 3.76 ± 0.41 g/dl ($p = 0.0001$) [2]. They suggested that the impact of HCV infection on nutritional status and inflammation may be a main cause of cardiovascular mortality in this population. Inflammation associated with chronic infections may contribute to the increased CVD death risk in dialysis individuals. In addition, multiple studies have shown that HCV is associated with liver steatosis, insulin resistance, and hypoadiponectinemia [18]. In addition to conventional cardiovascular risk factors in dialysis population such as hypertension, hypercholesterolemia, and hyperhomocysteinemia, HCV infection may be an important factor. This view is supported by the notion that traditional risk factors only partially explain the mortality excess in dialysis population [19].

The link between cardiovascular mortality and HCV infection in patients on long-term dialysis has been studied by Oyake et al. [20] using pulse-wave velocimeter measurements. They prospectively evaluated 94 dialysis patients (17 being HCV positive) by measurements of aortic stiffness (by carotid-femoral pulse wave velocity). Multiple logistic regression analysis found that mean blood pressure and HCV viremia (OR, 9.7, 95% CI, 1.18–81.19, $p < 0.05$) were significantly and independently associated with high PWV (≥10.0 m/s, mean). Kaplan-Meier survival curves for cerebrovascular and cardiovascular event-free rates indicated a highly significant difference between HCV RNA-positive or -negative patients on dialysis (log-rank test, $p < 0.05$). They suggested that HCV infection plays an atherogenic role through aggravation of metabolic syndrome and dyslipidemia.

According to the meta-analysis of observational studies reported above [12], the summary estimate for unadjusted RR of cardiovascular-related mortality was 0.95 (95% CI, 0.76–1.18), NS.

HCV: Survival and Quality of Life

It has been recently suggested that one of the mechanisms of increased mortality in HCV-positive patients is due to an impairment of quality of life (QOL). Several authors have noted that the QOL is diminished in dialysis population; also, HCV-infected individuals with intact kidney function have an impairment of QOL scores. However, the relationship between HCV infection and QOL among patients receiving long-term dialysis has been to date analyzed only by Afsar et al. [21]. They studied 165 patients on regular dialysis, 83 of whom being anti-HCV positive. They evaluated QOL by SF-36, a test which consists of 36 items, assigned to eight subscales, that can be summarized by a physical component summary score and mental component score (MCS). SF-36 has been commonly used and validated in CKD patients. There was an independent relationship between anti-HCV-positive status and reduced mental component summary score (B, –3.423, p = 0.016). No association with the physical component summary score was noted (NS). The presence of symptoms of depression might be one explanation – depression is frequent in patients with HCV as a reactive phenomenon related to the diagnosis ('labeling' effect) and concerns over long-term health. Depression may be secondary to symptoms such as fatigue and cognitive impairment that can be frequently observed in HCV-infected individuals. In addition, HD treatment is independently associated with an increased prevalence of depression, which in turn negatively affects health-related QOL. It remains unclear whether treatment of HCV in HD population can decrease mortality by improving QOL, irrespective of biological markers (i.e. liver histology or virologic features); thus, dialysis patients with advanced liver disease could still benefit from antiviral therapy in terms of QOL and therefore lowered mortality.

Natural History of HCV: Dialysis versus Non-Uremic Controls

Despite these data showing the adverse impact of anti-HCV serologic status on survival in the dialysis population, the course of HCV infection the dialysis population has not been fully characterized, although there is evidence promoting the notion of a difference in the natural history of chronic hepatitis C between dialysis and non-uremic populations. A severe clinical course of HCV-related liver disease seems unusual in most HD patients. Another distinctive feature is that antiviral therapy can be very effective in the minority of patients requiring such treatment. In a case-control study, Okuda and Yokosuka [22] gave the most important information to date. 189 patients with anti-HCV antibody were followed up for more than 4 years and compared with twice as many gender- and age-matched controls with chronic hepatitis C diagnosed in the same month as the case and followed up for comparable periods. The longest follow-up was 23 years in dialysis cases. No dialysis patients with chronic hepatitis C progressed to cirrhosis, whereas the disease progressed to cirrhosis in more than one quarter of the controls (62/228). These differences were highly significant ($p < 0.0001$).

Ishida et al. [23] found an incidence rate of HCC and cirrhosis of 1.8% (114/6,222) and 8.6% (536/6,242), respectively, in 314 dialysis units from Japan. These incidence rates appear much lower than those they attributed to normal adults, according to the medical literature (cirrhosis in 15–20%; HCC in 5–28%). Furthermore, the incidence rates of HCC and cirrhosis in patients who underwent HD therapy for more than 10 years were lower than in patients who had been on HD for less than 10 years: 0.5% (17/3,533) vs. 4.2% (79/1,870) and 6% (211/3,533) versus 13% (243/1,870), respectively. In view of the high risk of cancer in patients on maintenance HD, a very high incidence rate of HCC in dialysis patients with HCV had been postulated. The authors did not clarify the paradoxical phenomenon they found.

HCV Viral Load: Uremic versus Non-Uremic Controls

The relationship between HCV viral load and liver disease progression is currently a matter of debate. An increase in HCV RNA load by 8-fold or more compared with natural infection has been observed in various immunosuppressed populations, including liver or renal transplant recipients, and patients with HCV/HIV coinfection. The accelerated progression of HCV-related liver disease in these groups has been related, at least in part, to a high viral load. It remains unclear if these findings apply to dialysis patients with immune compromise due to chronic uremia. At least 5 cross-sectional studies [reviewed in 24] have concluded that the HCV load is lower in HCV-infected dialysis patients than in patients with chronic hepatitis C and intact kidney function, whereas at least 3 other studies [reviewed in 24] have failed to find any significant difference in the viral load between dialysis patients and non-uremic controls. Overall, the available information does not support an increase in HCV load in patients on maintenance HD despite the immune abnormalities related to uremia and the HD procedure per se.

There is a paucity of longitudinal studies of HCV virology during natural infection in chronic dialysis patients with HCV. Two prospective studies [24] have not reported differences in HCV viremia over time in patients on maintenance dialysis, but the short follow-up precluded definitive conclusions. In contrast, two prospective controlled trials with appropriate follow-up have given contrasting findings [24]. Furusyo et al. [25] found that HCV RNA levels were significantly lower in 98 HD patients (median, 0.4 mEq/ml) than in 228 non-uremic individuals (median, 3.0 mEq/ml; $p < 0.05$). Their prospective observations over 3 years revealed a significant decrease in HCV RNA levels in 47 HD patients with HCV genotype 1b (2.6 ± 0.7 vs. 1.8 ± 0.6 mEq/ml, $p = 0.0082$), whereas levels in 155 non-uremic subjects with genotype 1b did not decrease (5.7 ± 0.7 vs. 5.8 ± 0.6 mEq/ml, NS).

Histopathology of HCV-Related Liver Disease in Dialysis and Non-Uremic Controls

Evidence comparing liver biopsy findings between dialysis patients and non-uremic controls infected with HCV is limited. A large controlled study conducted by Cotler et al. [26] compared histology findings between renal transplant candidates (n = 46) and non-uremic individuals (n = 46) with chronic HCV. Study and control patients were well matched for age, gender, and race. All study patients with CKD had been on long-term dialysis. As already reported by other authors, aspartate aminotransferase and ALT were significantly lower in CKD patients than in the non-uremic controls. Patients with CKD had less inflammation, 3.5 (2.0–7.0) versus 6 (3.0–9.0), $p = 0.033$, and less bridging fibrosis or cirrhosis, 13% (6/46) versus 30% (14/46), $p = 0.043$, than controls. Similar observations were noted by other authors in another controlled study, although the small number of patients included (n = 20) prevented definitive conclusions [27]. Alric et al. [28] observed that Knodell score was similar between HCV-infected dialysis patients (n = 30) and control (non-transplanted and non-hemodialyzed) patients (n = 30), 5.14 ± 0.54 vs. 5.1 ± 0.3 (NS), although fibrosis progression/year was lower in HCV-infected HD patients than in controls, 0.11 (0.04–0.17) versus 0.17 (0.14–0.20), $p < 0.05$.

Kinetics of HCV Load during Hemodialysis

According to the data reported above, the question is why there is such a distinct difference in the natural history of chronic hepatitis C between dialysis and non-uremic patients. It is well known that liver injury caused by HCV is mainly through immunologic processes rather than due to a direct cythopathic activity of the virus. Current data suggest that many different immune disturbances occur in HD patients, and the lower immune competence of HD patients has been considered a possible cause of attenuated inflammatory reactions and reduced hepatocyte destruction caused by HCV.

It appears that the HD procedure per se can protect patients from a more aggressive course of HCV by reduction in the viral load. The mechanisms by which the HD procedure lowers HCV viremia remain largely speculative: the passage of viral particles into the dialysate [29, 30], the trapping of HCV on the surface of the dialysis membrane [31, 32], and an indirect host-mediated phenomenon have been cited. The latter hypothesis implicates the production of interferon-α [33], hepatocyte growth factors [27], or other cytokines with antiviral activities during the HD sessions.

Conclusions

HCV-related liver disease remains frequent in patients on long-term dialysis with an impact upon survival. Several lines of evidence support the concept that progression of HCV-related liver disease is probably slower than in HCV-infected individuals with intact kidney function, despite immune compromise due to uremia. Numerous mechanisms have been suggested to explain it, and it is possible that an indirect host-mediated mechanism could be involved. Clinical trials and experimental studies aimed at clarifying this issue are needed.

Acknowledgements

This work has been supported in part by the grant Project Glomerulonephritis. It is in memory of Pippo Neglia.

References

1 Kidney Disease Improving Global Outomes. KDIGO clinical practice guidelines for the prevention, diagnosis, evaluation and treatment of hepatitis C in chronic kidney disease. Kidney Int 2008;73:S1–S99.
2 Kalantar-Zadeh K, Kilpatrick R, McAllister C, Miller L, Daar S, Gjertson D, Kopple J, Greenland S: Hepatitis C virus and death risk in hemodialysis patients. J Am Soc Nephrol 2007;18:1584–1593.
3 Kalantar-Zadeh K, McAllister C, Miller LG: Clinical characteristics and mortality in hepatitis C-positive haemodialysis patients: a population based study. Nephrol Dial Transplant 2005;20:1662–1669.
4 Goral V, Simsek M, Mete N: Hepatic osteodystrophy and liver cirrhosis. World J Gastroenterol 2010;16:1639–1643.
5 Marcelli D, Stannard D, Conte F, Held P, Locatelli F, Port F: ESRD patient mortality with adjustment for comorbid conditions in Lombardy (Italy) versus the United States. Kidney Int 1996;50:1013–1018.
6 Fabrizi F, Martin P, Dixit V, Brezina M, Cole MJ, Gerosa S, Vinson S, Mousa M, Gitnick G: Quantitative assessment of HCV load in chronic haemodialysis patients: a cross-sectional survey. Nephron 1998;80:428–433.
7 Fabrizi F, De Vecchi A, Qureshi A, Aucella F, Lunghi G, Bruchfeld A, Bisegna S, Mangano S, Limido A, Vigilante D, Forcella M, Delli Carri P, Martin P: Gamma glutamyltranspeptidase activity and viral hepatitis in dialysis population. Int J Artif Organs 2007;30:6–15.
8 Stehman-Breen C, Emerson S, Gretch D, Johnson RJ: Risk of death among chronic dialysis patients infected with HCV. Am J Kidney Dis 1998;32:629–634.
9 Nakayama E, Akiba T, Marumo F, Sato C: Prognosis of anti-hepatitis C virus antibody-positive patients on regular hemodialysis therapy. J Am Soc Nephrol 2000;11:1896–1902.
10 Espinosa M, Martin-Malo A, Alvarez de Lara M, Alijama P: Risk of death and liver cirrhosis in anti-HCV positive long-term haemodialysis patients. Nephrol Dial Transplant 2001;16:1669–1674.

11 Di Napoli A, Pezzotti P, Di Lallo D, Petrosillo N, Trivelloni C, Di Giulio S, The Lazio Dialysis Registry: Epidemiology of hepatitis C virus among long-term dialysis patients: a 9-year study in an Italian registry. Am J Kidney Dis 2006;48:629–637.
12 Fabrizi F, Takkouche B, Lunghi G, Dixit V, Messa P, Martin P: The impact of hepatitis C virus infection on survival in dialysis patients: meta-analysis of observational studies. J Viral Hepat 2007;14:697–703.
13 Scott DR, Wong J, Spicer T, Dent H, Mensah F, McDonald S, Levy M: Adverse impact of hepatitis C virus infection on renal replacement therapy and renal transplant patients in Australia and New Zealand. Transplantation 2010;90:1165–1171.
14 Johnson D, Dent H, Yao Q, Tranaeus A, Huang C, Han D, Jha V, Wang T, Kawaguchi Y, Qian J: Frequencies of hepatitis B and C infections among haemodialysis and peritoneal dialysis patients in Asia-Pacific countries: analysis of registry data. Nephrol Dial Transplant 2009;24:1598–1603.
15 Santoro D, Mazzaglia G, Savica V, Li Vecchi M, Bellinghieri G: Hepatitis status and mortality in haemodialysis population. Ren Fail 2009;31:6–12.
16 Goodkin D, Bragg-Gresham J, Koenig K, et al: Association of comorbid conditions and mortality in hemodialysis patients in Europe, Japan and the United States: The dialysis outcomes, and practice patterns study (DOPPS). J Am Soc Nephrol 2003;14:3270–3277.
17 Wang SM, Liu H, Chou C, Huang C, Shih C, Chen W: Mortality in hepatitis C-positive patients treated with peritoneal dialysis. Perit Dial Intern 2008;28:183–187.
18 Petit JM, Minello A, Jooste V, et al: Decreased plasma adiponectin concentrations are closely related to steatosis in hepatitis C virus-infected patients. J Clin Endocrinol Metab 2005;90:2240–2243.
19 Kalantar-Zadeh K, Daar E, Eysselein V, Miller L: Hepatitis C infection in dialysis patients: a link to poor clinical outcome? Int Urol Nephrol 2007;39:247–259.
20 Oyake N, Shimada T, Murakami Y, Ishibashi Y, Satoh H, Suzuki K, Matsumori A, Oda T: Hepatitis C virus infection as a risk factor for increased aortic stiffness and cardiovascular events in dialysis patients. J Nephrol 2008;21:345–353.
21 Afsar B, Elsurer R, Sezer S, Ozdemir NF: Quality of life in haemodialysis patients: hepatitis C virus makes sense. Int Urol Nephrol 2009;41:1011–1019.
22 Okuda K, Yokosuka O: Natural history of chronic hepatitis C in patients on haemodialysis: case control study with 4–23 years of follow-up. World J Gastroenterol 2004;10:2209–2212.
23 Ishida H, Agishi T, Koyama I, Sawada T, Murakami T, Utsumi K, Tsuji K, Kawase T, Ishii Y, Ishimori I, kaneko I, Tojimbara T, Nakajima I, Mineshina M, Fuchinoue S, Yoshioka T: Hemodialysis paradox: survey on the incidence rate of hepatocellular carcinoma in anti-hepatitis virus C-antibody positive chronic haemodialysis patients. Artif Organs 2001;25:58–71.
24 Fabrizi F, Messa P, Martin P: Impact of haemodialysis therapy on hepatitis C virus infection: a deeper insight. Int J Artif Organs 2009;32:1–11.
25 Furusyo N, Hayashi J, Ariyama I, Sawayama Y, Etoh Y, Shigematsu M, Kashiwagi S: Maintenance haemodialysis decreases serum hepatitis C virus RNA levels in haemodialysis patients with chronic HCV infection. Am J Gastroenterol 2000;95:490–496.
26 Cotler S, Diaz G, Gundlapalli S, Jakate S, Chawla A, Mital D, Jensik S, Jensen DM: Characteristics of hepatitis C in renal transplant candidates. J Clin Gastroenterol 2002;35:191–195.
27 Rampino T, Arbustini E, Gregorini M, Guallini P, Libetta C, Maggio M, Ranghino A, Silini E, Soccio G, Dal Canton A: Haemodialysis prevents liver disease caused by hepatitis C virus: role of hepatocyte growth factor. Kidney Int 1999;56:2286–2291.
28 Alric L, Di Martino V, Selves J, et al: Long-term impact of renal transplantation on liver fibrosis during hepatitis C virus infection. Gastroenterology 2002;123:1494–1499.
29 Lombardi M, Cerrai T, Dattolo P, et al: Is the dialysis membrane a safe barrier against HCV infection? Nephrol Dial Transplant 1995;10:578–579.
30 Noiri E, Nakao A, Oya A, Fujta T, Kimura S: Hepatitis C virus in blood and dialysate in hemodialysis. Am J Kidney Dis 2001;37:38–42.

31 Mizuno M, Higuchi T, Yanai M, Kanmatsuse K, Esumi M: Dialysis-membrane-dependent reduction and adsorption of circulating C virus during haemodialysis. Nephron 2002;91:235–242.
32 Hayashi H, Okuda K, Yokosuka O, et al: Adsorption of hepatitis C virus particles onto the dialyzer membrane. Artif Organs 1997;21:1056–1059.
33 Badalamenti S, Catania A, Lunghi G, Covini G, Bredi E, Brancaccio D, Salvadori M, Como G, Ponticelli C, Graziani G: Changes in viremia and circulating interferon-alpha during haemodialysis in hepatitis C virus-positive patients: only coincidental phenomena? Am J Kidney Dis 2003;42:1–11.

Dr. Fabrizio Fabrizi
Divisione Nefrologica, Ospedale Maggiore, Pad. Croff
Via Commenda 15
IT–20122 Milano (Italy)
Tel. +39 2 55034553, E-Mail fabrizi@policlinico.mi.it

Morales JM (ed): Hepatitis C in Renal Disease, Hemodialysis and Transplantation.
Contrib Nephrol. Basel, Karger, 2012, vol 176, pp 54–65

Treatment of Hepatitis C in Dialysis Patients

Nuria Esforzado · Josep Maria Campistol

Department of Nephrology and Renal Transplantation, Hospital Clinic, Universitat de Barcelona, IDIBAPS, Barcelona, Spain

Abstract

Chronic infection with hepatitis C virus (HCV) is a major problem affecting a significant percentage of patients with end-stage renal failure (ESRD), with a negative impact on patient survival, and associated with accelerated progression of liver damage after undergoing a kidney transplant. After acute HCV infection, HCV infection becomes chronic in around 80% of patients and progresses to cirrhosis in about 20% of cases at 20 years of evolution. Treatments with interferon (IFN-α2a) and pegylated IFN are currently the only treatments that achieve a cure rate of about 30–45% of ESRD patients with chronic HCV infection. The combination with ribavirin (RBV) in the general population has improved the results, with a sustained virological response between 50% (genotype 1 and 4) and 80% (genotype 2 and 3); however, the poor tolerance to RBV in ESRD patients makes this treatment difficult in dialysis patients. Indication of antiviral treatment in HCV-positive patients on dialysis should be individualized. All HCV-positive candidates for kidney transplantation should be assessed to receive antiviral treatment before transplantation given the increased life expectancy compared to other HCV-positive patients on dialysis, the increased risk of progression of liver disease with immunosuppressive therapy and the inability to receive IFN therapy after renal transplantation.

Prevalence

Infection with hepatitis C virus (HCV) is the leading cause of chronic liver disease all over the world. According to the WHO report, over 170 million people worldwide are infected with HCV, and 3–4 million people are infected yearly. Despite the introduction of protective measures and universal screening of blood products, dialysis patients still have an increased risk of acquiring HCV infection. Prevalence of HCV infection in people with kidney failure is variable depending on geographic manufacturing area, and can be up to 88%. In Europe, the prevalence is between 3% in the UK and 44% in Poland [1]. According to the Spanish registry of kidney disease in 2007, from a total of 19,114 dialysis patients, 788 presented positive serology for HCV (4%).

Natural History of HCV Infection

The natural history of HCV infection is difficult to establish for various reasons [2]: (a) It is an asymptomatic disease in most cases; (b) normally, it is unknown where the infection has occurred, and (c) it is a disease with a long evolution and also occasionally coexists with other factors that may modify the course of liver disease, such as alcohol consumption, coinfection with HBV and/or coinfection with HIV. Unlike HBV infection, most cases of hepatitis C become chronic (56–86%), and once chronicity is established the viremia persists over time [2]. Progression to cirrhosis is usually silent and the diagnosis of cirrhosis is sometimes not made until the liver is sufficiently committed and the patient undergoes decompensation, which occurs usually years after diagnosis of cirrhosis. In Seeff's review [2] of a representative group of retrospective studies that analyzed the evolution of chronic HCV infection patients in a follow-up period between 9 and 29 years, between 17 and 55% of cases (42% average) progressed towards liver cirrhosis, between 1 and 23% developed hepatocellular carcinoma, and between 4 and 15% died of liver-related causes. However, prospective studies taking into account the evolution of HCV infection after a follow-up period between 8 and 16 years, the development of cirrhosis occurred between 7 and 16% (11% average), development hepatocellular carcinoma between 0.7 and 1.3%, and liver-related death between 1.3 and 3.7% [2]. Despite the discrepancies between the various studies, Seeff concluded that about 20% of adult patients with chronic HCV infection will develop liver cirrhosis 20 years after viral infection [2].

Given the long and slow course of HCV infection, and the short follow-up period in the population with end-stage renal failure (ESRD) on dialysis, HCV infection has a true impact of on mortality in these patients. A recent meta-analysis of the impact of HCV infection on mortality in 11,589 patients on dialysis, obtained from seven observational studies, defined an increased risk of mortality in HCV-positive patients (relative risk of mortality of 1.34, 95% CI 1.13–1.59, $p < 0.01$) [3], with the relative risk of death from liver disease of 5.89 (95% CI 1.93–17.99, $p < 0.001$) [3].

It is noteworthy that, after renal transplantation (RT), immunosuppressive therapy induces an increase in viral replication. In a review in our unit [unpubl. data] (fig. 1), viremia increased immediately after RT, reaching a peak between 6 and 12 months after RT.

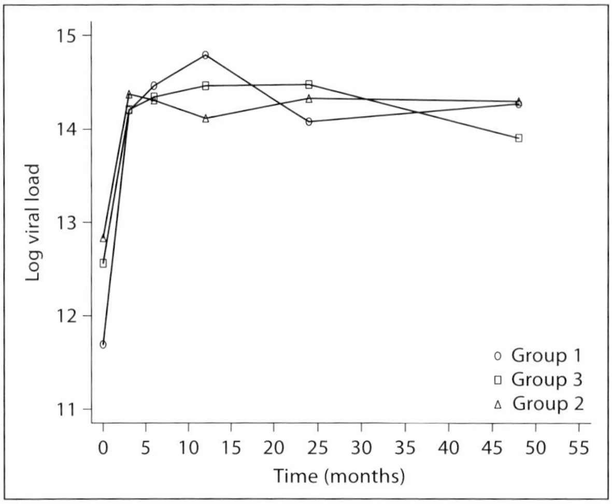

Fig. 1. Evolution of hepatitis C infection viremia after renal transplant. Mean viral load on a log-transformed scale in all patients. Group 1 = Cyclosporine/tacrolimus monotherapy (13 patients); group 2 = ATG/OKT3 induction (13 patients); group 3 = cyclosporine or tacrolimus, and mycophenolate mofetil (10 patients). Data from Esforzado and Campistol [unpubl.].

Differences in gender, genotype (GT), duration of infection, coinfection with other hepatotropic viruses and/or the concomitant use of potentially hepatotoxic drugs after transplantation may influence the clinical outcome of HCV liver disease. Thus, Fenning et al. [4] analyzing a homogeneous population in terms of gender, GT, source of infection and duration of HCV infection, observed a positive correlation between serum HCV-RNA and the degree of liver inflammation. On the other hand, according to the study by Zylberger et al. [5], comparing the hepatic progression determined by liver biopsy (median 7 years) in 28 RT patients, anti-HCV-positive patients and 28 anti-HCV-positive controls, histological damage was found in 70% of RT patients with HCV infection compared with 19% of anti-VHC-positive controls, and progression to liver cirrhosis at second liver biopsy (median 7 years) was 21% in the RT group and 3.6% in control group [5].

Treating HCV Infection in the General Population

In 1991, interferon-α (IFN-α) monotherapy for the treatment of chronic HCV infection was approved; however, sustained virological response (SVR) was achieved in less than 20% of patients. In 1998, the addition of ribavirin (RBV) was able to improve SVR rates to between 34 and 42%. In 2001, the availability of pegylated IFN (pegIFN) further increased the rates of SVR in approximately 50%.

The combination of RBV pegIFN with RBV achieved SVR rates of approximately 80% in individuals infected with GT2 or GT3 and 40–50% in persons infected with GT1 and GT4 [6].

To minimize treatment toxicity and achieve greater effectiveness, the duration of antiviral treatment is determined by the GT of HCV according to the initial response of the treatment. Thus, patients with GT1 and GT4 are usually treated for 48 weeks with pegIFN-α2a (180 μg/week) or pegIFN-α2b (1.5 μg/kg body weight per week) in combination with RBV 1,000–1,400 μg/day, while GT2 and GT3 patients are treated for 24 weeks with pegIFN-α2a or pegIFN-α2b and RBV. A rapid viral response at week 12 after starting treatment, with undetectable or ≥2 $\log_{10}$ decrease in serum HCV RNA is predictive of success after completing treatment [6]. Male gender, older age, higher body mass index, coinfections, insulin resistance and advanced liver disease contributed to a poorer response to treatment [6].

Justification for Treatment of HCV Infection in Dialysis Patients

Justification for the treatment of HCV infection in patients with ESRD on dialysis is based on the negative impact on overall mortality of these patients and liver-related mortality [3], as well as the accelerated progression of liver damage after undergoing RT [5], plus the increased risk of rejection and graft loss when given IFN after RT. The aim of this chapter is to review the results reported in the literature on the efficacy and tolerability of antiviral treatment in patients with ESRD treated with dialysis.

Results of Treatment of Chronic HCV Infection in Dialysis Patients: Literature Review

The goal of treatment for HCV infection in patients with chronic kidney disease is viral eradication in order to improve patient survival and the morbidity associated with HCV infection. Treatment options include standard IFN-α2a or IFN-pegIFN, alone or in combination with RBV.

The altered pharmacokinetics in these patients, the increased risk of drug-related toxicity and the need to undergo an RT complicates the management of antiviral therapy.

Several clinical trials evaluating IFN monotherapy have shown a higher SVR as well as a higher rate of treatment discontinuation related to adverse events in dialysis patients compared with patients with normal renal function.

Data on pegIFN alone or in combination with RBV are promising, but limited.

Table 1. Meta-analyses of IFN therapy in patients with ESRD

Reference	Year	Patients	Treatment	Doses	Treatment weeks	SVR %	Stop %
Fabrizi et al. [9]	2003	269	IFN-α	1.5–6.0 MU/day 3 times/week	12–48	37	17
Russo et al. [10]	2003	213	IFN-α	3.0–5.0 MU/day 3 times/week	24–48	33	30
Fabrizi et al. [11]	2008	645	IFN-α pegIFN-α	1.0–6.0 MU/day 3 times/week 135–180 μg/week (α2a) or 0.5–1.0 μg/kg/week (α2b)	8–48 48	39 31	19 27
Gordon et al. [7]	2008	546	INF-α pegIFN-α (±RBV)	1.0–6.0 MU/day 3 times/week 135–180 μg/week (α2a) or 0.5–1.0 μg/kg/week (α2b)	16–48 24–48	41 37	26 28
Gordon et al. [9]	2009	428	IFN-α	1.0–6.0 MU/day 3 times/week	16–48	45	26
Fabrizi et al. [17]	2010	254	pegIFN-α	135–180 μg/week (α2a) or 0.5–1.1 μg/kg/week (α2b)	24–48	33	23

Stop signifies treatment discontinuation.

Interferon Monotherapy

The SVR with conventional IFN-α2a monotherapy at doses of 3–6 MU three times weekly for 24–48 weeks was less than 20% in patients without ESRD with chronic HCV [6], while in patients with ESRD, according to what was observed in different meta-analysis [7–11], conventional treatment with IFN-α2a monotherapy achieved SVR in 33–45% of patients (table 1). However, the treatment dropout rate was between 17 and 30% of cases (table 1).

The recent meta-analysis by Gordon et al. [8] on the response to IFN treatment in 428 hemodialysis patients with chronic HCV infection obtained from 22 prospective studies showed an SVR in 45% of cases, giving better response when treatment was administered for at least 6 months at a dose of at least three million units of IFN three times a week, when treatment was completed, when the patient was on low viral load, when the patient was female, and when the patient achieved a negative viremia at the first 3 months of starting treatment. The greatest response to IFN in dialysis patients with chronic HCV infection compared to the general population may be due to pharmacokinetic alterations of IFN, with a lower renal clearance and higher serum concentrations of IFN in dialysis patients [12], although other patient-related factors and viruses may contribute to the response of the treatment.

The discontinuation of IFN therapy in hemodialysis patients is variable with an average of 26% in the study of Gordon et al. [8], but varies between 0 and 50% in the analyzed studies. Although Gordon et al. [8] found no link between high doses of IFN and discontinuation of treatment, they found an increase in the development of adverse effects (influenza-like symptoms or anemia) at higher doses. According to Gordon et al. [8], the negative conversion of viremia in the first 3 months of treatment is associated with an SVR in 67% of cases, while only 25% of patients who did not achieve negative viral load in the first 3 months achieved an SVR [8]. Thus, in accordance with other authors, the negative conversion of the viral load in the first 3 months is a strong predictor of SVR at the end of treatment [13].

Pegylated Interferon

The efficacy and tolerability of pegIFN monotherapy in patients with ESRD is not well established. In patients without ESRD with chronic HCV infection, the rate of SVR and dropout rate with pegIFN alone (pegIFN-α2a at a dose of 180 μg/week or pegIFN-α2b at doses of 0.5–1.5 μg/kg/week) administered for 48 weeks are 18–39 and 3–7%, respectively [14, 15]. In patients with creatinine clearance <30 ml/min, AUC and C_{max} of IFN increased by 90% compared to healthy volunteers, while the lifetime increased to 40% compared to controls; moreover, the hemodialysis pegIFN affected the clearance [16].

The response to pegIFN monotherapy is comparable to that obtained with conventional IFN. Based on three meta-analyses including a total of 457 patients, SVR was achieved in 31–37% of patients with a dropout rate of 23–28% (table 1) [7, 11, 17]. However, in a recent study, 50 dialysis patients with HCV infection were randomized to receive IFN-α2a or pegIFN, and patients receiving pegIFN-α2a tended to have higher SVR than those who received IFN-α2a (48 vs. 20%, p = 0.07) [13]. Using multivariate analysis, treatment with pegIFN-α2a (p = 0.02) and HCV RNA viral load prior to treatment <800,000 IU/ml (p = 0.007) were independent predictors of SVR. In addition, patients who received pegIFN-α2a had a significantly lower rate of discontinuation of treatment than those receiving conventional IFN-α2a (0 vs. 20%, p = 0.04) [13].

Interferon and Ribavirin

The combination of IFN and RBV (1,000–1,400 mg/day) improves the response to treatment with IFN and pegIFN in patients without renal failure [6]. Treatment with peg-IFN and RBV can eradicate HCV infection in 40–50% of patients infected with HCV GT 1 or 4 and about 80% of patients infected with GT 2 or 3 [6]. However, in patients on dialysis, the RBV is generally not recommended because of the risk of hemolytic anemia. Since the RBV is eliminated by the kidney, an overdose can result in severe anemia, so it is not recommended for use when the creatinine clearance is <50 ml/min [18]. Several studies using low doses of RBV from 200 mg 3 times per week to 400 mg daily, combined with high-dose IFN and erythropoietin managed to treat patients with ESRD and HCV infection. The response was achieved in 17–67% of cases with an incidence of discontinuation of up to 33% [19, 20] (table 2).

Table 2. Treatment with IFN and RBV in patients with ESRD

Study	Year	Patients	Treatment	Treatment, weeks	SVR %	Stop %
IFN + RBV						
Bruchfeld et al. [19]	2001	6	IFN-α2b + RBV	28	17	33
Mousa et al. [20]	2004	20	IFN-α + RBV	24 48	67 36	0 0
Pgylated IFN + RBV						
Bruchfeld et al. [21]	2006	6	pegIFN-α2a or 2b + RBV	24[1]–48[2]	50	33
Rendina et al. [22]	2007	35	pegIFN-α2a + RBV	24[3]–48[4]	97	14
Carriero et al. [23]	2008	14	pegIFN-α2a + RBV	48	29	71
Van Leusen et al. [24]	2008	7	pegIFN-α2a + RBV	24[1]–48[2]	71	0
Hakim et al. [25]	2009	15	pegIFN-α2a + RBV	48	7	33
Liu et al. [26]	2009	35	pegIFN-α2a + RBV	24[1]–48[4]	60	17

[1] GT2.
[2] GT1 and GT4.
[3] Non-GT1.
[4] GT1.

Few studies have examined the efficacy and safety of low-dose pegIFN RBV in patients with ESRD [21–24]. High doses of erythropoietin are needed to maintain adequate doses of RBV during treatment [21, 22]; however, the response is very variable, with an SVR between 7 and 97% and a dropout rate of up to 71% [23] (table 2).

Treatment of Acute HCV Infection in Dialysis Patients

In ESRD patients on dialysis with acute HCV infection, treatment with conventional IFN or pegIFN is effective and relatively well tolerated [27]. Monitoring of serum levels of HCV RNA in the first 16 weeks of acute infection is useful to avoid performing unnecessary treatments in a small percentage of patients who will present a spontaneous cure of hepatitis C [28]. In a recent study that included 42 patients with acute HCV hepatitis, 7 patients (16.6%) became spontaneously HCV RNA negative in the first 16 weeks of infection, while the remaining 35 patients (83%) did not spontaneously become HCV RNA negative; after the first 16 weeks under observation, they

HCV RNA-positive patients
Therapy is widely accepted • Age 18 years or older, and • HCV RNA positive in serum, and • Liver biopsy showing chronic hepatitis with significant fibrosis • Compensated liver disease • Acceptable hematological and biochemical indices • Willing to be treated and to adhere to treatment requirements, and • No contraindications
Therapy should be individualized • Failed prior treatment (non respondents and relapsers) either IFN with or without RBV or pegINF monotherapy • Current users of illicit drugs or alcohol but willing to participate in a substance abuse program or alcohol support program. Candidates should be abstinent for a minimum period of 6 months • Liver biopsy evidence of either no or mild fibrosis • Acute hepatitis C • Coinfection with HIV • Under 18 years of age • Decompensated cirrhosis • Liver transplant recipients • Chronic renal disease
Therapy is currently contraindicated • Major uncontrolled depressive illness • Solid organ transplant (renal, heart or lung) • Autoimmune hepatitis or other autoimmune condition known to be exacerbated by IFN and RBV • Untreated thyroid disease • Pregnant or unwilling to comply with adequate contraception • Severe concurrent medical disease such as severe hypertension, heart failure, significant coronary heart disease, poorly controlled diabetes, chronic obstructive pulmonary disease • Age less than 2 years • Known hypersensitivity to drugs used to treat HCV

Fig. 2. Indications, contraindications, and individualization of treatment of HCV infection (KDIGO and AASLD recommendations) [29, 30].

were treated with IFN-α2a at a dose of 135 μg/week for 24 weeks, and 88% achieved an SVR [28].

Accordingly, both the KDIGO [29] and AASLD [30] guidelines recommend waiting between 8 weeks and a maximum of 12 weeks from the onset of infection to rule out spontaneous resolution of infection.

Recommendations for the Treatment of HCV Infection in Dialysis Patients

Indications and contraindications for the treatment of HCV infection are resumed in figure 2. In chronic renal disease patients, therapy to eradicate HCV infection should be individualized (fig. 3).

KDIGO guidelines [29] recommend treatment with conventional IFN (2a or 2b) 3 MU three times weekly or reduced doses of pegIFN 2a 135 μg/week or 2b

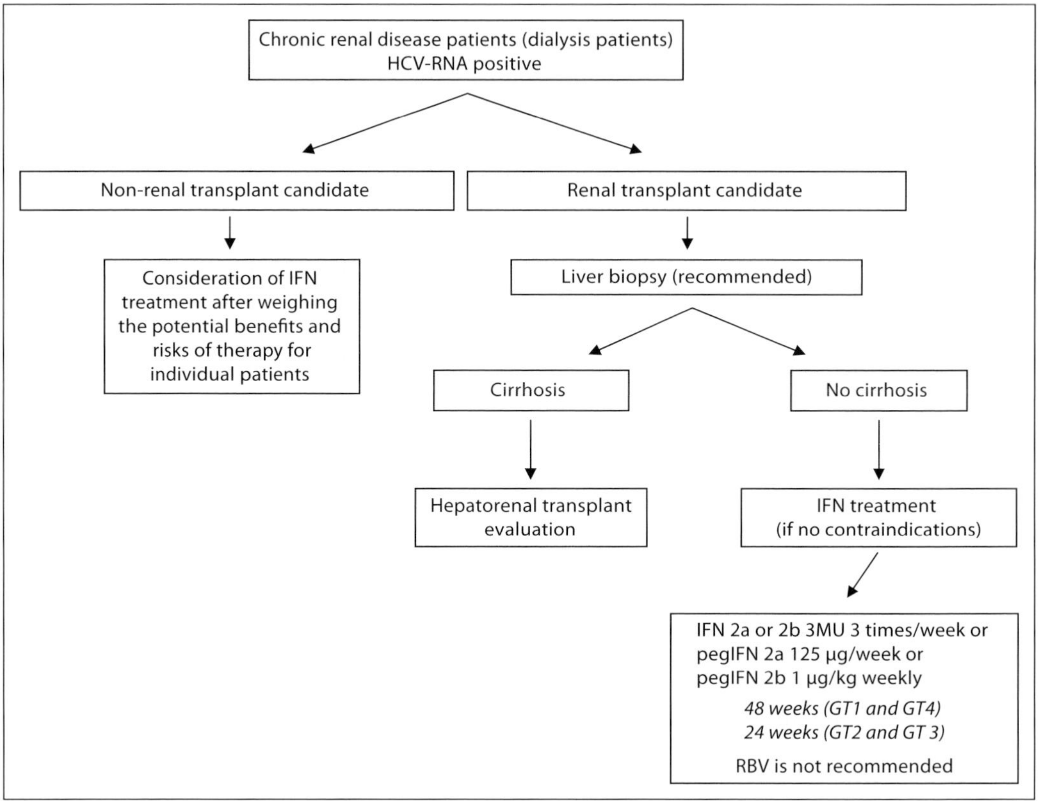

Fig. 3. Individualization of treatment of HCV infection in dialysis patients.

1 µg/kg weekly; however, the indication for treatment should be based on the potential benefits and risks of treatment and life expectancy, the possibility of receiving a kidney transplant patient and comorbidities [29]. The duration of treatment is 48 weeks for the HCV infection with GT1 and GT4 if a rapid viral load decrease is observed at 12 weeks (>2 log viral titer in fall), and 24 weeks for the HCV infection GT2 and GT3 [29]. RBV is not recommended in patients on dialysis but can be used in combination with low-dose IFN with a strict monitoring of anemia [30]. The decision to perform liver biopsy should be individualized based on patient's clinical situation, the need for treatment and the need to establish the severity of liver disease [30]. According to the KDIGO guidelines, treatment should be recommended to all HCV-positive RT candidates since life expectancy in this group of patients is higher than in the other patients on dialysis due to the increased risk of progression of liver disease related to immunosuppressive therapy and the risk of renal graft dysfunction when given IFN after transplantation [29].

Interferon Side Effects

The toxicity associated with therapy represents a major obstacle facing both the current treatment in patients with ESRD and in the general population, with an impact on quality of life of patients leading to dose reduction in 35–42% and sometimes to discontinuation of treatment (30% of patients) [31]. The main side effects include flu-like symptoms (e.g. fever, fatigue, headache, myalgia and arthralgia), blood disorders (e.g. anemia and neutropenia), and neuropsychiatric symptoms (e.g. depression and anxiety) [31].

In summary, HCV infection is associated with increased mortality in patients with ESRD on dialysis. Despite the introduction of protective measures and universal screening of blood products, dialysis patients still have an increased risk of acquiring HCV infection.

Acute HCV infection in dialysis patients, treatment with IFN, pegylated or conventional, has a high response rate above 80%.

In chronic HCV infection, about one third of dialysis patients treated with IFN monotherapy achieve an SVR, with no differences in values between conventional and pegylated IFN, respectively. However, the dropout rate is high due to frequent adverse effects.

The combination of pegIFN with RBV may be an alternative in ESRD patients with HCV infection as long as low doses of RBV are used as well as a close monitoring of anemia is made. A low HCV RNA load before starting treatment and rapid clearance of the virus are factors that predict SVR, both in those receiving IFN as well as those receiving pegIFN.

Indication of antiviral treatment in HCV-positive patients on dialysis should be individualized. All HCV-positive RT candidates should be assessed for treatment with IFN before transplantation due to the increased life expectancy compared to other HCV-positive patients on dialysis, the increased risk of progression of liver disease after RT and the association of treatment with IFN with renal graft dysfunction after transplantation.

References

1 Jadoul M, Poignet JL, Geddes C, Locatelli F, Medin C, Krajewska M, Barril G, Scheuermann E, Sonkodi S, Goubau P, HCV Collaborative Group: The changing epidemiology of hepatitis C virus (HCV) infection in haemodialysis: European multicentre study. Nephrol Dial Transplant 2004;19:904–909.

2 Seeff LB: Natural history of chronic hepatitis C. Hepatology 2002;36:S35–S46.

3 Fabrizi F, Takkouche B, Lunghi G, Dixit V, Messa P, Martin P: The impact of hepatitis C virus infection on survival in dialysis patients: meta-analysis of observational studies. J Viral Hepat 2007;14:697–703.

4 Fenning L, Kenny E, Sheehan M, Cannon B, Whelton M, O'Conneh J, Collins JK, Shanahan F: Viral load and clinicopathological features of chronic hepatitis C (1b) in a homogeneus patient population. Hepatology 1999;29:904–907.

5 Zylberberg H, Nalpas B, Carnot F, Skhiri H, Fontaine H, Legendre C, Kreis H, Bréchot C, Pol S: Severe evolution of chronic hepatitis C in renal transplantation: a case control study. Nephrol Dial Transplant 2002;17:129–133.
6 TenCate V, Sainz Jr B, Cotler SJ, Uprichard SL: Potential treatment options and future research to increase hepatitis C virus treatment response rate. Hepat Med 2010;2:125–145.
7 Gordon CE, Uhlig K, Lau J, Schmid CH, Levey AS, Wong JB: Interferon treatment in hemodialysis patients with chronic hepatitis C virus infection: a systematic review of the literature and meta-analysis of treatment efficacy and harms. Am J Kidney Dis 2008;51:263–277.
8 Gordon CE, Uhlig K, Lau J, Schmid CH, Levey AS, Wong JB: Interferon for hepatitis C virus in hemodialysis – an individual patient meta-analysis of factors associated with sustained virological response. Clin J Am Soc Nephrol 2009;4:1449–1458.
9 Fabrizi F, Dulai G, Dixit V, Bunnapradist S, Martin P: Meta-analysis: interferon for the treatment of chronic hepatitis C in dialysis patients. Aliment Pharmacol Ther 2003;18:1071–1081.
10 Russo MW, Goldsweig CD, Jacobson IM, Brown RS Jr: Interferon monotherapy for dialysis patients with chronic hepatitis C: an analysis of the literature on efficacy and safety. Am J Gastroenterol 2003;98:1610–1615.
11 Fabrizi F, Dixit V, Messa P, Martin P: Interferon monotherapy of chronic hepatitis C in dialysis patients: meta-analysis of clinical trials. J Viral Hepat 2008;15:79–88.
12 Rostaing L, Chatelut E, Payen JL, Izopet J, Thalamas C, Ton-That H, Pascal JP, Durand D, Canal P: Pharmacokinetics of alphaIFN-2b in chronic hepatitis C virus patients undergoing chronic hemodialysis or with normal renal function: clinical implications. J Am Soc Nephrol 1998;9:2344–2348.
13 Liu CH, Liang CC, Lin JW, Chen SI, Tsai HB, Chang CS, Hung PH, Kao JH, Liu CJ, Lai MY, Chen JH, Chen PJ, Kao JH, Chen DS: Pegylated interferon alpha-2a versus standard interferon alpha-2a for treatment-naive dialysis patients with chronic hepatitis C: a randomised study. Gut 2008;57:525–530.
14 Zeuzem S, Feinman SV, Rasenack J, Heathcote EJ, Lai MY, Gane E, O'Grady J, Reichen J, Diago M, Lin A, Hoffman J, Brunda MJ: Peginterferon alfa-2a in patients with chronic hepatitis C. N Engl J Med 2000;343:1666–1672.
15 Lindsay KL, Trepo C, Heintges T, Shiffman ML, Gordon SC, Hoefs JC, Schiff ER, Goodman ZD, Laughlin M, Yao R, Albrecht JK, Hepatitis Interventional Therapy Group: A randomized, double-blind trial comparing pegylated interferon alfa-2b to interferon alfa-2b as initial treatment for chronic hepatitis C. Hepatology 2001;34:395–403.
16 Gupta SK, Pittenger AL, Swan SK, Marbury TC, Tobillo E, Batra V, Sack M, Glue P, Jacobs S, Affrime M: Single-dose pharmacokinetics and safety of pegylated interferon-alpha2b in patients with chronic renal dysfunction. J Clin Pharmacol 2002;42:1109–1115.
17 Fabrizi F, Dixit V, Messa P, Martin P: Pegylated interferon monotherapy of chronic hepatitis C in dialysis patients: meta-analysis of clinical trials. J Med Virol 2010;82:768–775.
18 Brochot E, Castelain J, Duverlie G, Capron D, Nguyen-Khac E, François C: Ribavirin monitoring in chronic hepatitis C therapy: anemia versus efficacy. Antiviral Ther 2010;15:687–695.
19 Bruchfeld A, Stahle L, Andersson J, Schvarcz R: Ribavirin treatment in dialysis patients with chronic hepatitis C virus infection – a pilot study. J Viral Hepat 2001;8:287–292.
20 Mousa DH, Abdalla AH, Al-Shoail G, Al-Sulaiman MH, Al-Hawas FA, Al-Khader AA: Alpha-interferon with ribavirin in the treatment of hemodialysis patients with hepatitis C. Transplant Proc 2004;36:1831–1834.
21 Bruchfeld A, Lindahl K, Reichard O, Carlsson T, Schvarcz R: Pegylated interferon and ribavirin treatment for hepatitis C in haemodialysis patients. J Viral Hepat 2006;13:316–321.
22 Rendina M, Schena A, Castellaneta NM, Losito F, Amoruso AC, Stallone G, Schena FP, Di Leo A, Francavilla A: The treatment of chronic hepatitis C with peginterferon alfa-2a (40 kDa) plus ribavirin in haemodialysed patients awaiting renal transplant. J Hepatol 2007;46:768–774.

23 Carriero D, Fabrizi F, Uriel AJ, Park J, Martin P, Dieterich DT: Treatment of dialysis patients with chronic hepatitis C using pegylated interferon and low-dose ribavirin. Int J Artif Organs 2008;31:295–302.
24 Van Leusen R, Adang RP, de Vries RA, Cnossen TT, Konings CJ, Schalm SW, Tan AC: Pegylated interferon alfa-2a (40 kD) and ribavirin in haemodialysis patients with chronic hepatitis C. Nephrol Dial Transplant 2008;23:721–725.
25 Hakim W, Sheikh S, Inayat I, Caldwell C, Smith D, Lorber M, Friedman A, Jain D, Bia M, Formica R, Mehal W: HCV response in patients with end stage renal disease treated with combination pegylated interferon alpha-2a and ribavirin. J Clin Gastroenterol 2009;43:477–481.
26 Liu CH, Liang CC, Liu CJ, Tsai HB, Hung PH, Hsu SJ, Chen SI, Lin JW, Lai MY, Chen JH, Chen PJ, Chen DS, Kao JH: Pegylated interferon alfa-2a plus low dose ribavirin for the retreatment of dialysis chronic hepatitis C patients who relapsed from prior interferon monotherapy. Gut 2009;58:314–316.
27 Liu CH, Kao JH: Treatment of hepatitis C virus infection in patients with end-stage renal disease. J Gastroenterol Hepatol 2011;26:228–239.
28 Liu CH, Liang CC, Liu CJ, Lin JW, Chen SI, Hung PH, Tsai HB, Lai MY, Chen PJ, Chen DS, Kao JH: Pegylated interferon alfa-2a monotherapy for hemodialysis patients with acute hepatitis C. Clin Infect Dis 2010;51:541–549.
29 Kidney Disease: Improving Global Outcomes (KDIGO): KDIGO clinical practice guidelines for the prevention, diagnosis, evaluation, and treatment of hepatitis C in chronic kidney disease. Kidney Int Suppl 2008;109:S1–S99.
30 Ghany MG, Strader B, Thomas DL, Seeff LB: Diagnosis, management and treatment of hepatitis C: an update. Hepatology 2009;49:1335–1374.
31 Sulkowski CMS, Cooper C, Hunyady B, Jia J, Ogurtsov P, Peck-Radosavljevic M, Shiffman ML, Yurdaydin C, Dalgard O: Management of adverse effects of Peg-IFN and ribavirin therapy for hepatitis C. Nat Rev Gastroeneterol Hepatol 2011;8:212–223.

Dra. Nuria Esforzado
Renal Transplant Unit, Hospital Clinic Barcelona
C/Villarroel 170
ES–08036 Barcelona (Spain)
Tel. +34 932275444, E-Mail nesforza@clinic.ub.es

Morales JM (ed): Hepatitis C in Renal Disease, Hemodialysis and Transplantation.
Contrib Nephrol. Basel, Karger, 2012, vol 176, pp 66–76

Selection and Management of Hepatitis C Virus-Infected Patients for the Kidney Transplant Waiting List

David Roth[a] · Roy Bloom[b]

[a]Division of Nephrology and Hypertension, University of Miami Miller School of Medicine, Miami, Fla., and [b]Division of Nephrology, University of Pennsylvania School of Medicine, Philadelphia, Pa., USA

Abstract

Hepatitis C virus (HCV) infection has been demonstrated to be present in a significant number of ESRD patients, and infection with this virus has been shown to have a detrimental impact on patient survival in both the dialysis and transplant patient populations. Studies have shown that 10–25% of pre-kidney transplant candidates have advanced liver injury with stage 3 or 4 disease (cirrhosis) when biopsied during the pretransplant evaluation. To identify those patients in whom a more extensive workup is required, all transplant candidates should be initially screened for anti-HCV antibody and/or active viremia using nucleic acid testing depending on the prevalence of HCV in the community. Although efforts have been directed at finding a reliable noninvasive marker of advanced liver disease in this patient population, liver biopsy remains the gold standard and should be obtained during the pretransplant evaluation in all patients determined to have active HCV infection. There is general agreement that patients with established or decompensated cirrhosis should be referred to the liver transplant team for consideration of combined liver-kidney transplantation. Patients on the kidney transplant waiting list should be monitored on a regular basis to identify those who might have progressive liver disease. This is especially relevant in an era when waiting times at some centers approach 5–7 years. There is no consensus on whether the pretransplant patient with active HCV viremia should be treated with antiviral agents prior to transplant. There is some largely anecdotal evidence that inducing a sustained virological response prior to transplant might lessen the risk of developing posttransplant diabetes and immune complex-mediated glomerular disease in the allograft. Whereas there is good evidence that the majority of patients achieving a sustained virological response prior to transplant do not relapse following the introduction of immunosuppression, there are limited data as to whether this has a positive impact on the progression of liver injury. Several studies have demonstrated that the use of interferon in the posttransplant setting is associated with an increased risk of allograft rejection; thus, any efforts to eradicate HCV should be focused on the pretransplant period. In summary, a thorough screening process to identify HCV infection in the pre-kidney transplant candidate, including the staging of liver disease in those determined to have viremia, is necessary so that the most appropriate treatment plan can be developed for each patient.

Screening and Evaluation of Kidney Transplant Candidates for Hepatitis C Virus Infection

Kidney transplantation has been demonstrated to offer a survival advantage for hepatitis C virus (HCV)-infected patients when compared to remaining on dialysis [1–4]. Nevertheless, HCV infection has been shown to impart an adverse impact on patient survival amongst both dialysis and transplant patients [5, 6]. This increased risk is attributable to a higher incidence of both hepatic and nonhepatic complications. In addition, HCV-infected patients on the waiting list have an increased mortality when compared to noninfected patients [2]. In this context, it is imperative that transplant centers carefully screen for HCV infection during the pretransplant evaluation. Patients determined to be infected must have a thorough evaluation to determine their suitability for kidney transplantation. In this chapter, we discuss the evaluation and waiting list management of these patients, including considerations for cirrhotics, as well as treatment strategies that can be employed for wait-listed individuals.

Characteristics of Wait-Listed Kidney Transplant Candidates with HCV Infection

Among kidney recipients, the prevalence of chronic HCV infection prior to transplantation has been documented to range from 7 to 40%, with wide geographic and demographic variation [7, 8]. Risk factors for HCV infection in this population include duration of ESRD, prior transplantation, black race as well as a history of hepatitis B virus coinfection and prior substance abuse [9]. Studies have also demonstrated that HCV infection in patients with ESRD is associated with underlying diabetes mellitus [2, 9]. Diabetes mellitus is present in about 30% of HCV-infected kidney candidates aged 30–50 years, and the prevalence increases in an age-dependent manner thereafter, reaching 63% among elderly candidates [2]. Diabetes mellitus remains a leading cause of ESRD and contributes to the increased comorbidity burden in the kidney transplant population with HCV infection.

Screening Tests

Studies have demonstrated that up to 25% of those determined to have active HCV infection have advanced stages of liver fibrosis on liver biopsy [4, 10–14]. These patients usually have well-compensated liver disease and would otherwise not be suspected of harboring serious liver injury. As a consequence of this often undiagnosed burden of liver disease, it is essential that all patients being considered for kidney transplantation have a thorough screening to determine if HCV infection is present. As recommended by the KDIGO Workgroup [15], patients living in geographical regions of the world with a low prevalence of HCV infection should have initial testing with EIA. Patients found to be anti-HCV positive by EIA should have follow-up confirmation using nuclear acid testing (NAT) to document viremia. In high HCV prevalence settings, initial testing with NAT should be the first line screening since a negative EIA cannot reliably exclude the presence of infection (KDIGO guideline 1.1.2; fig. 1).

Establishing Liver Disease Severity

In keeping with the KDIGO HCV guidelines, we believe that a baseline liver biopsy should be performed in all HCV-infected kidney transplant candidates with persistent viremia. Liver biopsy is needed to ascertain the extent of liver injury and damage, and may impact on both the prognosis and management of patients. Reasons supporting pretransplant liver biopsy in this population include (a) the inability of noninvasive studies to predict the histological severity of liver disease, (b) the fact that up to 25% of HCV-infected potential kidney candidates have bridging fibrosis or cirrhosis that may be associated with worse posttransplant outcomes, and (c) the possibility that liver disease may progress after transplant and that liver biopsy may help guide treatment to prevent this.

Whereas liver biopsy remains the 'gold standard' to establish the extent of liver injury in HCV-infected patients, there have been efforts to identify noninvasive markers of liver disease that might allow transplant physicians to avoid the need for a liver biopsy prior to listing an HCV-infected patient for kidney transplant. This has been fueled by the concern that ESRD patients present a higher risk for complications related to percutaneous liver biopsy compared to patients with normal kidney function [16]. This is largely focused on issues of impaired platelet function in the ESRD patient [17]. In fact, studies have shown that a percutaneous liver biopsy can be safely performed in ESRD patients without undue risk of bleeding, and current recommendations do not support the need for using the transjugular route [4, 18].

Attempts at finding a reliable noninvasive marker to establish the severity of liver disease in the HCV-infected kidney transplant candidate have been

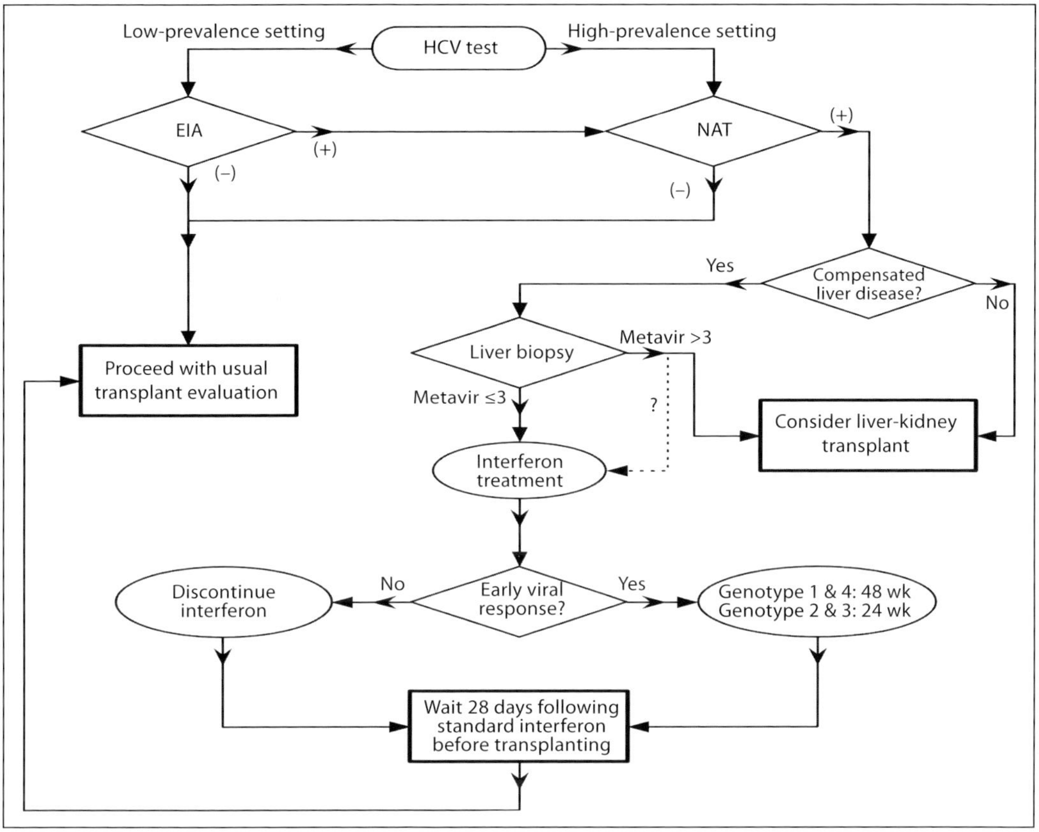

Fig. 1. Screening and treatment of HCV infection in the kidney transplant candidate. Reprinted from *Kidney International* with permission of Nature Publishing Group.

largely unsuccessful. Liver transaminases have been shown to be lower in dialysis patients than HCV-infected patients with normal kidney function and are not reliable for making a decision on who should be biopsied or in predicting the severity of liver disease [19]. Measurement of the platelet count and aspartate aminotransferase was used by Schiavon et al. [20] to derive the AST to platelet count ratio (APRI). In this study, both the AST and the platelet count were independent predictors of significant fibrosis on biopsy. They also found that an APRI <0.40 accurately identified patients with stage 0 or 1 disease with a negative predictive ratio of 93%. Less impressive results were obtained in the prediction of significant fibrosis with a positive predictive value of only 66% for the presence of significant fibrosis in patients with a high APRI score. There are very limited data available on the use of transient elastography (Fibroscan) to assess the extent of liver fibrosis in patients with kidney disease. One study evaluated the use of Fibroscan in HCV-infected kidney transplant recipients and found that the scores seemed to correlate well with the degree of fibrosis on liver biopsy [21]. There are no comparable studies in kidney transplant candidates.

Several groups have reported the results of pre transplant liver biopsies in ESRD patients being evaluated for kidney transplantation [4, 10–14]. A quality liver biopsy of at least 2 cm in length and containing 45 portal zones is required for adequate Metavir scoring [22–24]. In the study by Roth et al. [4], 207 patients were biopsied as part of the pre-kidney transplant evaluation of HCV RNA-positive patients. In this analysis, 80% of the patients had stage 0/1 liver disease, 6% were stage 3 and 4% had stage 4 fibrosis (cirrhosis). None of these patients had clinical evidence of advanced liver disease (ascites, encephalopathy, etc.) when referred to the center for kidney transplantation. Other studies have reported similar findings with 10–25% of patients having stage 3 or 4 disease [10–14]. Patients with stage 3 and possibly very early stage 4 disease can be considered for kidney-alone transplantation; however, a careful assessment of the increased risk must be taken into consideration. This is a growing issue as an increasing number of HCV-infected CKD patients with well-compensated cirrhosis considered 'too healthy' to qualify for liver transplantation present for evaluation for a kidney transplant alone.

The risks associated with kidney transplantation in cirrhotic patients include both increased perioperative morbidity and mortality related to limited reserve and nutritional status, increased susceptibility to infectious and metabolic complications, as well as inferior longer term survival. A recent retrospective analysis of single center data from the Mayo Clinic examined postoperative mortality in 772 patients with cirrhosis undergoing major surgery. Thirty-day mortality was 5.7% in patients with the least severe cirrhosis as defined by the MELD score [25]. Since serum creatinine is an important component of this metric, the utility of MELD specifically in kidney transplant patients is unknown. Moreover, since only about 20% of patients in this study had 'viral' hepatitis, it is not known whether these findings are generalizable to a solely HCV-associated cirrhotic population.

A recent consensus conference on simultaneous liver-kidney transplantation (SLKT), co-sponsored by the American Society of Transplantation, the American Society of Transplant Surgeons, the American Society of Nephrology as well as the United Network for Organ Sharing proposed using portal hypertension criteria in well-compensated cirrhotics to determine listing for SLKT versus kidney alone [26]. The specific consensus recommendation is that patients with a Wedge Hepatic Vein Pressure <10 mm Hg be listed for a kidney transplant alone, although this remains to be validated in practice. In our own programs, we additionally include the absence of varices on endoscopy, as well as a platelet count above $120 \times 10^3/\mu l$ as criteria to consider for listing for a kidney alone. There are no definitive studies that have evaluated long-term posttransplant outcomes in HCV-infected kidney recipients with cirrhosis on pretransplant liver biopsy. In a single-center series, survival at 10 years after transplant was only 26% among the few patients that had pretransplant cirrhosis [27]. There is general agreement that patients with established or decompensated cirrhosis should be referred to the liver transplant team for consideration of combined liver-kidney transplantation.

In summary, although there continues to be interest in finding a noninvasive method to assess the extent of liver fibrosis in HCV-infected kidney transplant candidates, there are as yet no tests that provide the accuracy and reliability of information obtained from a liver biopsy. In this context, the KDIGO Workgroup recommended that a percutaneous liver biopsy be obtained in all HCV-infected patients being considered for kidney transplantation [15].

Management of HCV-Infected Patients on the Kidney Waiting List

Most transplant centers have been screening for HCV infection as part of the pre-kidney transplant evaluation for many years, and as a consequence the majority of patients on kidney transplant waiting lists have already been tested for HCV and determined to be a suitable candidate for kidney-alone transplant. In the context of a steady increase in waiting times for a deceased donor kidney transplant, with some areas of the US approaching 5–7 years, it is imperative that a protocol be in place for the ongoing surveillance of the HCV-infected patient on the kidney waiting list to ensure their continued suitability for kidney transplantation.

Patients on the waiting list who were never tested for the presence of HCV infection prior to listing should be screened for anti-HCV antibodies by EIA (with confirmation of positive results by NAT) in regions with a low prevalence of infection and directly with NAT in high prevalence settings. Patients who are found to have a positive NAT should be placed on hold status and referred to a hepatologist for evaluation and possible treatment [15].

It was the opinion of the KDIGO Workgroup [15] that patients who were known to be HCV infected prior to transplant and had achieved a sustained virological response (SVR) with antiviral therapy should be tested at least annually with NAT to confirm the durability of the SVR. Patients with relapse should be placed on hold status and referred to a hepatologist for consideration of retreatment. Patients who were listed while still viremic should have an annual evaluation to ensure that the liver disease has not progressed. In the study of Roth et al. [4], there were 13 patients who had a repeat liver biopsy while still on the transplant waiting list. In this group, 8/13 (62%) patients demonstrated interval worsening of the liver histology in sharp contrast to the results from follow-up liver biopsies obtained after transplant where only 7/31 (23%) showed interval worsening. Progression of hepatitis C-related liver disease has been demonstrated by other authors in wait-listed dialysis patients [28, 29]. It was the

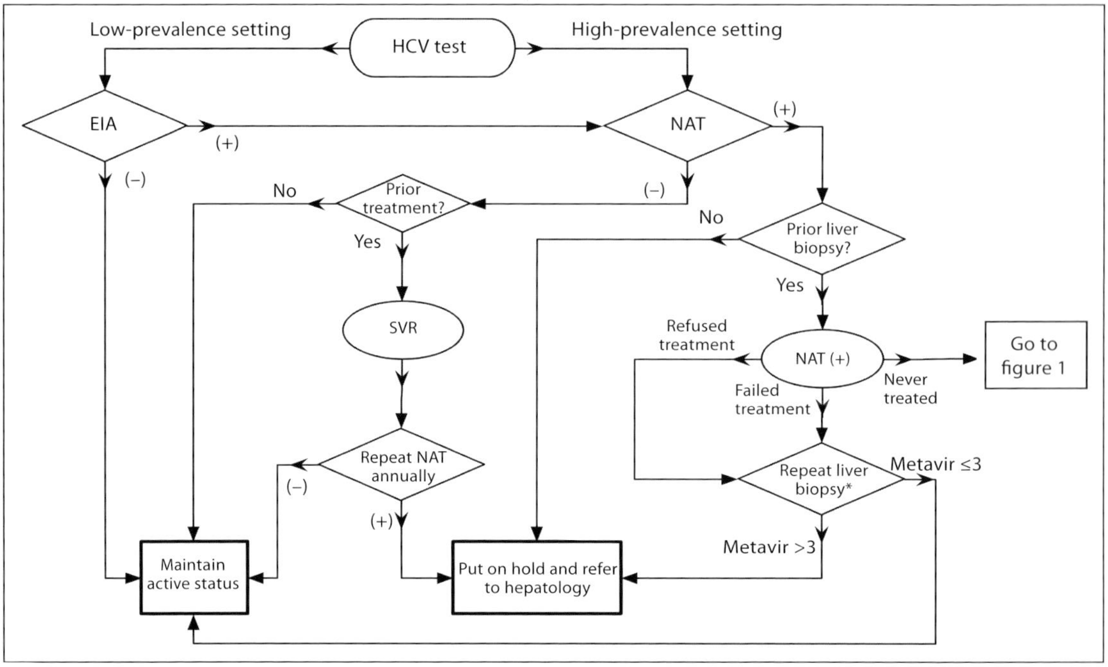

Fig. 2. Management of the wait-listed pretransplant candidate. Reprinted from *Kidney International* with permission of Nature Publishing Group.

opinion of the KDIGO Workgroup [15] that patients whose pretransplant liver biopsy showed Metavir stage 1 or 2 fibrosis should have a repeat liver biopsy every 5 years, while those with stage 3 fibrosis should be watched more carefully and thus rebiopsied in 3 years. Patients whose liver disease has progressed to early or established cirrhosis should be removed from the kidney list and referred to the liver team for consideration of simultaneous liver-kidney transplant (fig. 2).

The death rate for patients on kidney transplant waiting lists in the US is approximately 6–7%, with cardiovascular disease being the leading contributor to this mortality. It has been demonstrated that HCV-infected patients with CKD and in the general population have an increased prevalence of diabetes mellitus [30, 31]. To further examine this relationship in patients awaiting kidney transplantation, Bloom, et al. [2] reported data from a single-center study of HCV-infected kidney candidates who were on the kidney waiting list. Of interest, the prevalence of diabetes was significantly higher amongst the HCV-infected cohort. Moreover, in a Cox regression model in which the usual clinical variables were entered, only diabetes was associated with an increased risk for death (HR: 2.17, 95% CI: 1.1–4.1; $p = 0.02$). Of note, liver disease was not predictive of mortality in the model.

As emphasized earlier, in an era where waiting times for a kidney often exceed 5 years, careful and frequent monitoring of the HCV-infected patient on the waiting list must be part of the protocol for these patients. Evaluation of listed patients must account for the possibility of worsening liver disease that might preclude kidney-alone transplantation. In the study by Bloom et al. [2], death on the list was the primary reason that HCV-infected patients were delisted, with liver disease being far less frequent. In this context, consideration must be given to providing robust surveillance for cardiovascular disease considering the high prevalence of diabetes in this cohort of patients and the enormous burden of cardiovascular disease that is known to be present in the CKD population.

Treatment of HCV in Kidney Transplant Candidates

Progress has been made over the past 1–2 decades in the treatment of HCV infection in the general population. A detailed discussion of specific antiviral treatment for HCV-infected CKD patients is provided elsewhere in this book. As already alluded to, HCV-infected kidney recipients have worse patient and graft survival as a result of the development, and/or progression, of both hepatic as well as extrahepatic complications. Achieving an SVR, the standard measure of successful HCV therapy, prior to kidney transplantation is a desirable goal for several reasons.

First, although standard interferon (IFN) and pegylated IFN result in SVR rates of only 45 and 37%, respectively [32], this response is usually durable for those patients in whom an SVR can be attained. Gordon et al. [33] have recently performed a systematic review of 31 studies of IFN-based treatment of patients with ESRD. By extracting patient level data on 45 patients that achieved SVR and were subsequently transplanted, they were able to demonstrate that the probability of remaining with an undetectable HCV viral load was 95% by 48 months after transplant. However, no detailed information was provided in this study regarding liver histology or clinical progression of liver disease after transplantation.

A second rationale for trying to attain an SVR prior to transplant is to prevent the development of extrahepatic complications after transplant. A few retrospective studies have reported that a durable SVR obtained before transplant was associated with no cases of new diabetes mellitus after transplantation, as well as improved insulin sensitivity [34, 35]. Moreover, Cruzado et al. [36] performed a small controlled trial where they demonstrated that wait-listed kidney candidates in whom SVR was obtained prior to transplantation had a significantly lower incidence of HCV-associated glomerulopathy after transplant.

A final important consideration favoring administration of IFN-based therapies before transplantation is related to the concern that this antiviral therapy is associated with an increased risk of acute rejection when administered in the post-kidney transplant setting [discussed in 14]. This complication, reported to occur in 40–100% of IFN-treated kidney recipients, has been attributed to the immunomodulatory properties of the therapy, including upregulation of several cytokine genes and HLA antigens [37]. Based on this risk, KDIGO guidelines further recommend that patients should not be transplanted while they are receiving IFN and should be in an 'on-hold' status until the therapy is completed. The risk–benefit ratio of delaying transplantation in the hope of achieving SVR with prolonged administration of IFN is unknown.

Conclusions

Kidney transplantation is the treatment of choice for HCV-infected patients with advanced CKD. This population has a significantly greater comorbidity burden than their uninfected counterparts. Besides the obvious association with liver disease, patients with HCV also have a higher rate of underlying diabetes mellitus, with risk for its attendant complications. A thorough assessment of liver disease severity and other comorbidities is therefore recommended as part of the initial evaluation process, while listed patients require frequent and careful reevaluation to ensure that they remain viable transplant candidates. Conventional IFN-based therapies administered prior to transplant may reduce the risk of posttransplant HCV-related complications.

References

1 Pereira BJ, Natov SN, Bouthot BA, Murthy BVR, Ruthhazer R, Schmid CH, Levey AS: Effects of hepatitis C infection and renal transplantation on survival in end-stage renal disease. The New England Organ Bank Hepatitis C Study Group. Kidney Int 1998;53:1374–1381.

2 Bloom RD, Sayer G, Fa K, Constantinescu S, Abt P, Reddy R: Outcome of hepatitis C virus-infected kidney transplant candidates who remain on the waiting list. Am J Transplant 2005;5:139–144.

3 Knoll GA, Tankersley MR, Lee JY, Julian BA, Curtis JJ: The impact of renal transplantation on survival in hepatitis C-positive end-stage renal disease patients. Am J Kidney Dis 1997;29:608–614.

4 Roth D, Gaynor J, Reddy R, Ciancio G, Sageshima J, Kupin W, Guerra G, Chen L, Burke G: Outcomes in hepatitis C patients before and after kidney transplantation. J Am Soc Nephrol 2011;22:1152–1160.

5 Fabrizi F, Martin P, Dixit V, Bunnapradist S, Dulai G: Meta-analysis: effect of hepatitis C virus infection on mortality in dialysis. Aliment Pharmacol Ther 2004;20:1271–1277.

6 Fabrizi F, Martin P, Dixit V, Bunnapradist S, Dulai G: Hepatitis C virus antibody status and survival after renal transplantation: meta-analysis of observational studies. Am J Transplant 2005;5:1452–1461.

7 Vosnides GG: Hepatitis C in renal transplantation. Kidney Int 1997;52:834–861.

8 Hanafusa T, Ichikawa Y, Kishikawa H, et al: Retrospective study on the impact of hepatitis C virus infection on kidney transplant patients over 20 years. Transplantation 1998;66:471–476.
9 Fissell RB, Bragg-Gresham JL, Woods JD, et al: Patterns of hepatitis C prevalence and seroconversion in hemodialysis units from three continents: the DOPPS. Kidney Int 2004;65:2335–2342.
10 Martin P, Carter D, Fabrizi F, Dixit V, Conrad AJ, Artinian L, Peacock V, Han S, Wilkinson A, Lassman CR, Danovitch G: Histopathological features of hepatitis C in renal transplant candidates. Transplantation 2000;69:1479–1484.
11 Sterling RK, Sanyal AJ, Luketic VA, Stravitz RT, King AL, Post AB, Mills AS, Contros MJ, Schiffman ML: Chronic hepatitis C infection in patients with end stage renal disease: characterization of liver histology and viral load in patients awaiting renal transplantation. Am J Gastroenterol 1999;94:3576–3582.
12 Caramelo C, Ortiz A, Aguilera B, Porres JC, Navas S, Marriott E, Alberola MC, Alamo C, Galera A, Garron MP: Liver disease patterns in hemodialysis patients with antibodies to hepatitis C virus. Am J Kidney Dis 1993;22:822–828.
13 Glicklich D, Thung SN, Kapoian T, Tellis V, Reinus JF: Comparison of clinical features and liver histology in hepatitis C-positive dialysis patients and renal transplant recipients. Am J Gastroenterol 1999;94:159–163.
14 Pol S, Romeo R, Zins B, Driss F, Lebkiri B, Garnot F, Berthelot P, Brechot C: Hepatitis C virus RNA in anti-HCV positive hemodialyzed patients: significance and therapeutic implications. Kidney Int 1993;44:1097–2000.
15 Kidney Disease: Improving Global Outcomes. KDIGO Clinical Practice Guidelines for the Prevention, Diagnosis, Evaluation and Treatment of Hepatitis C in Chronic Kidney Disease. Kidney Int 2008;73(suppl 109):S1–S99.
16 Cotler SJ, Diaz G, Gundiapalli S, et al: Characteristics of hepatitis C in renal transplant candidates. J Clin Gastroenterol 2002;35:191–195.
17 Brophy DF, Martin EJ, Carr SL, et al: The effect of uremia on platelet contractile force, clot elastin modulus and bleeding time in hemodialysis patients. Thromb Res 2007;119:723–729.
18 Pawa S, Ehrinpreis M, Mutchnick M, Janisse J, Dhar R, Siddiqui F: Percutaneous liver biopsy is safe in chronic hepatitis C patients with end stage renal disease. Clin Gastroenterol Hepatol 2007;5:1316–1320.
19 Furusyo N, Hayashi J, Kanamoto-Tanaka Y, et al: Liver damage in hemodialysis patients with hepatitis C virus viremia: a prospective 10-year study. Dig Dis Sci 2000;45:2221–2228.
20 Schiavon L, Schiavon J, Filho RJ, Sampaio J, Lanzoni V, Silva A, Ferraz M: Simple blood tests as noninvasive markers of liver fibrosis in hemodialysis patients with chronic hepatitis C virus infection. Hepatology 2007;46:307–314.
21 Munoz R, Ramirez E, Fernandez I, Martin A, Romero M, Romero E, Dominguez-Gil B, Hernandez A, Morales E, Andres A, Castellano G, Morales JM: Correlation between fibroscan, liver biopsy and clinical liver function in patients with hepatitis C virus infection after renal transplantation. Trans Proc 2009;41:2425–2426.
22 Bravo AA, Sheth SG, Chopra S: Liver biopsy. N Engl J Med 2001;344:495–500.
23 Regev A, Berho M, Jeffers LJ, et al: Sampling error and intraobserver variation in liver biopsy in patients with chronic HCV infection. Am J Gastroenterol 2002;97:2614–2618.
24 Sherlock S: The liver in Digestive Disease Week 1997. J Hepatol 1997;27:938–940.
25 Teh SH, Nagorney DM, Stevens SR, et al: Risk factors for mortality after surgery in patients with cirrhosis. Gastroenterology 2007;132:1261–1269.
26 Eason JD, Gonwa TA, Davis CL, Sung RS, Gerber D, Bloom RD: Proceedings of Consensus Conference on Simultaneous Liver Kidney Transplantation (SLK). Am J Transplant 2008;8:2243–2251.
27 Mathurin P, Mouquet C, Poynard T, et al: Impact of hepatitis B and C virus on kidney transplantation outcome. Hepatology 1999;29:257–263.

28 Pereira BJ, Natov SN, Bouthot BA, et al: Effects of hepatitis C infection and renal transplantation on survival in end-stage renal disease. The New England Organ Bank Hepatitis C Study Group. Kidney Int 1998;53:1374–1381.
29 Nakayama E, Akiba T, Marumo F, et al: Prognosis of anti-hepatitis C virus antibody-positive patients on regular hemodialysis therapy. J Am Soc Nephrol 2000;11:1896–1902.
30 Lecube A, Hernandez C, Genesca J, et al: High prevalence of glucose abnormalities in patients with hepatitis C virus infection: a multivariate analysis considering the liver injury. Diabetes Care 2004;27:1171–1175.
31 Mehta SH, Brancati FL, Sulkowski MS, et al: Prevalence of type 2 diabetes mellitus among persons with hepatitis C virus infection in the United States. Ann Intern Med 2000;133:592–599.
32 Gordon CE, Uhlig K, Lau J, Schmid CH, Levey AS, Wong JB: Interferon treatment in hemodialysis patients with chronic hepatitis C virus infection: a systematic review of the literature and meta-analysis of treatment efficacy and harms. Am J Kidney Dis 2008;51:263–277.
33 Gordon CE, Uhlig K, Schmid CH, Levey AS, Wong JB: Long-term viral negativity after interferon for chronic hepatitis C virus infection in hemodialysis. Clin J Am Soc Nephrol 2011;6:2226–2234.
34 Delgado-Borrego A, Casson D, Schoenfeld D, et al: Hepatitis C virus is independently associated with increased insulin resistance after liver transplantation. Transplantation 2004;77:703–710.
35 Kamar N, Toupance O, Buchler M, et al: Evidence that clearance of hepatitis C virus RNA after alpha-interferon therapy in dialysis patients is sustained after renal transplantation. J Am Soc Nephrol 2003;14:2092–2098.
36 Cruzado JM, Casanovas-Taltavull T, Torras J, Baliellas C, Gil-Vernet S, Grinyo JM: Pretransplant interferon prevents hepatitis C virus-associated glomerulonephritis in renal allografts by HCV-RNA clearance. Am J Transplant 2003;3:357–360.
37 Baid S, Tolkoff-Rubin N, Saidman S, et al: Acute humoral rejection in hepatitis C-infected renal transplant recipients receiving antiviral therapy. Am J Transplant 2003;3:74–78.

David Roth, MD
Division of Nephrology and Hypertension
1120 NW 14 Street
Suite 360-R (R126)
Miami, FL 33136 (USA)

Morales JM (ed): Hepatitis C in Renal Disease, Hemodialysis and Transplantation.
Contrib Nephrol. Basel, Karger, 2012, vol 176, pp 77–86

Kidney Transplantation in the Patient with Hepatitis C Virus Infection

Jose M. Morales[a] · Roy Bloom[b] · David Roth[c]

[a]Nephrology Department, Hospital 12 de Octubre, Madrid, Spain; [b]University of Pennsylvania Medical Center, Philadelphia, Pa., and [c]Division of Nephrology and Hypertension, Department of Medicine, University of Miami Miller School of Medicine, Miami, Fla., USA

Abstract

Liver disease is an important comorbidity following kidney transplantation, and hepatitis C virus (HCV) infection has been demonstrated to be the leading cause of this complication. Anti-HCV-positive kidney transplant recipients have a higher risk for developing proteinuria, chronic rejection, infections, glomerulonephritis and new-onset diabetes after transplantation (NODAT). Together with progressive liver disease in some patients, these complications all contribute to inferior patient and graft survival rates observed in anti-HCV-positive patients when compared to their uninfected counterparts. The increased mortality in the anti-HCV-positive cohort is largely as a result of a higher incidence of cardiovascular disease, liver disease and infections. HCV can also contribute to the development of some extrahepatic neoplasias, such as posttransplant lymphoproliferative disease. HCV infection is also an independent risk factor for graft loss, likely contributed to by the development of NODAT, chronic rejection/transplant glomerulopathy and HCV-related glomerulonephritis. Despite the increased comorbidities associated with kidney transplant in the HCV-infected patient, transplantation offers the best long-term outcomes for the end-stage renal disease patient with HCV infection. Finally, several interventions designed to minimize the potentially adverse consequences of HCV infection should be considered in the posttransplant setting. Adjustment of immunosuppression and careful follow-up in the outpatient clinic for early detection of proteinuria, renal insufficiency, infection, NODAT, neoplasia or worsening of liver disease are important components of the posttransplant care of the patient with HCV infection.

Hepatitis C virus (HCV) infection is currently the main cause of chronic liver disease in kidney transplant recipients [1–5]. The prevalence of HCV infection in patients with CKD exceeds that in the general population [5], and HCV is not only causative of kidney disease but also contributes to an increased morbidity and mortality in patients with established end-stage renal disease (ESRD) [5].

The impact of HCV infection on kidney transplantation starts with the consequences of this infection while the patient is still on the transplant waiting list. As the prevalence of HCV infection in dialysis patients has decreased [5], so too has it decreased among patients on the waiting list and therefore among those with a functioning allograft. In fact, a collaborative study performed in Spain that retrospectively reviewed the outcome of kidney transplant patients during the years 1990, 1994 and 1998 reported a progressive and significant decline in the prevalence of anti-HCV antibodies from 29.5 to 19 and 10%, respectively [6]. As will be discussed in more detail in this chapter, kidney transplantation has been demonstrated to be the preferred treatment for HCV-infected patients with ESRD, although graft and patient survival are lower compared to uninfected patients [1–5].

This chapter will review the literature with respect to the influence of HCV infection on acute rejection (AR), infection and extrahepatic neoplasia. Secondly, the impact of HCV infection on patient and graft survival will be summarized and finally several recommendations to minimize and/or prevent the consequences of HCV infection in kidney transplant patients will also be provided.

Influence of HCV Infection on Rejection, Infection and Neoplasia

Glomerulonephritis and new-onset diabetes after transplantation (NODAT; see chapter 11) are frequent complications associated with the presence of HCV infection in the kidney transplant recipient [2–5]. This infection can also influence the incidence of AR, serious infections as well as the development of certain extrahepatic neoplasias [7–9]. In this context, it is likely that these complications contribute either directly or indirectly to the diminished patient survival observed among HCV-infected kidney transplant recipients.

Acute Rejection in Anti-HCV-Positive Patients

There are conflicting data pertaining to the influence of HCV infection on the incidence of AR following kidney transplantation. Corell et al. [10] reported that HCV infection induced a state of immune deficiency in kidney recipients based on a reduction in the rate of naive T helper lymphocytes and an alteration in the proliferative responses of T lymphocytes to mitogens. These alterations would be expected to translate into a decreased incidence of AR, which in fact has been described by some groups. Roth et al. [11] recently reported an AR rate of 14.5% in HCV-infected patients followed over a 20-year period.

In contrast, other series found a similar or even greater incidence of AR in anti-HCV-positive patients [5]. To this point, the same factors associated with a higher risk of acquiring HCV infection in the pretransplant period are similar to those placing the patient at an increased risk for AR. Clinical variables such as time on dialysis, previous transplants and the number of blood transfusions are all risk factors for HCV infection in kidney transplant patients. At the same time, these factors are also associated with an increased immunological risk profile for the patient. This could possibly explain why anti-HCV-positive kidney transplant patients exhibit a higher than expected risk of AR in some series despite a decrease in immune responsiveness associated with viral infection. In one report, Forman et al. [12] observed a higher incidence of antibody-mediated AR in a series of 354 anti-HCV-positive kidney transplant patients. When adjusted for a PRA of >20%, HCV infection was no longer an independent risk factor for the development of antibody-mediated AR. In another study, patients transplanted between 1990 and 1994 were compared with a cohort of patients transplanted between 1998 and 2002 [13]. The incidence of AR was higher in anti-HCV-positive patients transplanted in the more modern era compared to the older cohort (25 vs. 20.6%, $p = 0.01$). This observation could possibly be explained by the increased number of second transplant patients and highly sensitized recipients in the anti-HCV-positive group [13].

It is therefore reasonable to consider whether the immune-mediated damage sustained by the allograft in anti-HCV-positive kidney recipients is related to the coexistence of immunological high risk, and whether this could account for the lower death-censored graft survival that has been reported in this population. As discussed above, there are conflicting data regarding the incidence of AR among anti-HCV-positive patients. However, solid clinical information is lacking with regard to the incidence of subclinical AR in these patients. In a series of 435 kidney transplant patients who underwent protocol biopsies in the first 6 months after transplantation, subclinical AR with chronic allograft nephropathy (CAN) and HCV infection were both independent risk factors for graft loss [14]. This would suggest that the immunological damage of the graft does not on its own explain the higher incidence of graft loss in anti-HCV-positive kidney transplant patients.

Infections in Anti-HCV-Positive Patients

Infection has been identified to be one of the leading causes of death in HCV-infected kidney transplant patients. In fact, it was reported many years ago that patients with what was then described as non-A non-B hepatitis had 'a marked increase of life-threatening extrahepatic complications' [15]. The increased risk for serious infectious complications has been confirmed in anti-HCV-positive patients, who had an increased frequency of postoperative infections and life-threatening infections of the central nervous system, lungs and blood stream than recipients without HCV infection [16]. The most recent experience in a prospective multicenter study from 2003 to 2005 found no differences between anti-HCV-positive and -negative recipients in the overall incidence of infection, although anti-HCV-positive recipients had a higher cumulative incidence of bloodstream and upper urinary tract infections. In this analysis, anti-HCV status was an independent risk factor for bloodstream infection only [17]. Another recent report demonstrated that HCV infection was an important risk factor for the development of tuberculosis in kidney recipients [18]. The reasons underlying the increased susceptibility to infection are not entirely clear. Several studies have demonstrated a strong association between diabetes in the pre- and posttransplant setting and increased patient mortality [19–21]. It is very possible that the diabetic comorbidity burden of HCV infection predisposes kidney recipients to other infectious complications, especially in the milieu of immunosuppression.

Intuitively, it would seem that this increased propensity for serious infection in the HCV-infected kidney transplant recipient would translate into an adverse impact on patient and graft survival. In this context, Roth et al. [11] recently reported that the increased death rate from infection can be demonstrated within the first 6 months after transplant, a period when the impact of induction and early higher doses of maintenance immunosuppressive therapy is greatest. Taken together, these data would suggest that a cautious approach to immunosuppression should be used for the HCV-infected kidney transplant recipient. The increased risk of infection-related morbidity and mortality must be balanced against that associated with the higher immunological risk profile of this population. The optimal immunosuppressive regimen for the HCV-infected patient has not been determined; however, understanding the risks present in this cohort of patients is essential for obtaining improved patient outcomes.

HCV Infection and Posttransplant Extrahepatic Neoplasia

The occurrence of posttransplant lymphoproliferative disorder (PTLD) has been recently associated with HCV infection in several analyses. In a study from Italy of over 1,000 liver, heart and kidney recipients, the overall prevalence of PTLD was 1.4% (0.8% in kidney transplant patients) and significantly higher in anti-HCV-positive (3.6%) compared to anti-HCV-negative patients (1.2%) [7]. In the French Registry of PTLD occurring in kidney allograft recipients, HCV infection was demonstrated to be an independent risk factor for mortality [8]. In the American Registry that included over 66,000 transplant recipients, 160 (0.24%) developed multiple myeloma with an increased prevalence of HCV infection in the myeloma subset, suggesting for the first time a possible association between HCV infection and this hematologic malignancy [9]. In addition, data from Australia and New Zealand showed that malignancy was the third leading cause of death in anti-HCV-positive patients, exceeding even that from liver disease [22]. Although these preliminary data must be confirmed in additional studies, they suggest that HCV infection could play a role in the pathogenesis of PTLD and other hematological neoplasias. In this context, the link between HCV infection and posttransplant malignancies observed in all these registry data analyses, while striking, requires further validation. Until then, we suggest close clinical surveillance for malignancy in the HCV-infected allograft recipient.

Impact of HCV Infection on Patient and Graft Survival after Kidney Transplantation

Influence of HCV Infection on Patient Survival

Numerous studies have demonstrated that HCV-infected kidney transplant recipients have inferior survival when compared to patients without evidence of HCV infection [5]. Most of the studies that were able to show this adverse impact on survival were those that examined data from patients who were >10 years after transplantation [5, 23–26]. Studies with a shorter posttransplant interval generally demonstrated no difference in outcomes between anti-HCV-positive and -negative recipients [5, 23]. It is important to note that all of these studies were retrospective in design and relied on ELISA assays to classify patients as 'infected' without the results of more accurate nucleic acid testing. Moreover, pretransplant liver biopsies were not performed in most of these studies, thereby precluding evaluation of the contribution of preexisting liver damage to the adverse posttransplant outcomes. Nevertheless, the results were consistent across a number of studies including a large number of patients from different countries. In a meta-analysis by Fabrizi et al. [27] of 8 clinical trials encompassing 6,365 patients, the authors were able to show a relative risk (RR) of 1.79 (95% CI 1.57–2.03) for mortality associated with HCV infection. The increased mortality was partly explained by an increase in liver-related death.

Although these results are of interest, the more relevant clinical question is what form of kidney replacement therapy is optimal for patients who are infected with HCV. Are the best outcomes obtained by having the patient remain on dialysis or should they be referred for kidney transplantation? Although the answer to this important question will never be obtained from a randomized, prospective study, there are a number of important publications that have provided important insight into this issue to help guide clinicians and patients when making this decision. Knoll et al. [28] first reported that there was a significantly lower mortality in anti-HCV-positive patients who were transplanted vs. those who remained on dialysis. This was followed by a report from Pereira et al. [29] who demonstrated that anti-HCV-positive patients receiving a kidney transplant had an RR of death of 0.31 in the 7–48 months posttransplant period compared to patients remaining on the waiting list for a transplant. Bloom et al. [19] also showed that transplanted patients infected with HCV had a lower mortality with transplantation compared to those remaining on the waiting list. In a recent report, Roth et al. [11] analyzed the effect of transplant status as a time-dependent covariate on the hazard rate for death in a group of 175 listed transplant candidates with documented HCV infection. Whereas the hazard ratio (HR) of death was 2.51 (95% CI 1.12–5.66; $p = 0.03$) in the first 6 months after transplant, this figure dropped to 0.32 (95% CI 0.17–0.62; $p < 0.001$) during the posttransplant period of 7–84 months. These results are all consistent in demonstrating that the survival advantage conferred by transplantation in the general ESRD [30] is still present in the subset of HCV-infected ESRD patients.

Taken together, whereas it appears that HCV infection confers an increased risk for mortality compared to a non-infected comparator group of kidney recipients, it is clear that transplantation remains the renal replacement therapy of choice for the HCV-infected ESRD patient assuming that the patient does not have advanced liver injury on pretransplant liver biopsy. Furthermore, the increased risk of infection-related death after transplant that has been demonstrated in several studies requires further analyses to better understand if certain immunosuppressive medications are better or worse for kidney transplant recipients.

Influence of HCV Infection on Graft Survival

Several studies have compared graft survival between anti-HCV-positive and -negative groups [5]. The majority of these reports were retrospective in design. In one study, Morales et al. [6] compared 488 anti-HCV-positive patients with 2,877 seronegative recipients and found an adjusted RR for graft loss of 1.53 ($p < 0.05$). Similar outcomes were reported by Bruchfield et al. [31] and Gentil et al. [32]. In a recently published study using the Australian and New Zealand Dialysis and Transplant Registry, Scott et al. [22] found that graft survival at 5 years was worse in the anti-HCV-positive cohort with an adjusted HR of 1.71 ($p < 0.001$) for graft failure. The cause of graft loss in the anti-HCV-positive group was significantly more likely to be due to glomerulonephritis (aHR = 2.71) and chronic allograft nephropathty (aHR = 1.87). In contrast, one prospective [33] and two retrospective studies have reported a decrease in graft loss in HCV-positive recipients, although these results did not reach statistical significance [20, 34].

In the meta-analysis by Fabrizi et al. [27], the presence of anti-HCV antibodies was an independent and significant factor for graft failure (RR 1.56, 95% CI 1.35–1.80, $p = 0.019$) in four of the eight studies included in the analysis. It is important to note that these four significant studies included the majority of the patients used for this meta-analysis.

Several HCV-related complications may contribute to decreased death-censored graft survival after renal transplantation, including the development of proteinuria due to CAN/IFTA and/or HCV-associated glomerulonephritis and NODAT. Hestin et al. [35] identified HCV infection as an independent risk factor for proteinuria after transplantation. The histopathological study in patients with proteinuria demonstrated a nonsignificant greater frequency of de novo glomerular lesions in anti-HCV-positive patients. Notably, CAN was the most frequent lesion, showing that nearly half of anti-HCV-positive patients had transplant glomerulopathy (TG). Some investigators have suggested a possible association between HCV infection and TG, though this has not been a consistent observation [2, 3]. In this context, Cosio et al. [36] found that the prevalence of anti-HCV antibodies was significantly higher in patients with TG than in those without this lesion (1.9 vs. 33%, respectively). The authors postulated that HCV infection, either directly, indirectly, or by inducing the release of cytokines such as interferon, may induce endothelial cell injury that eventually expresses itself clinically as TG.

In summary, long-term patient and graft survival rates are lower in anti-HCV-positive compared to anti-HCV-negative recipients. The higher risk of mortality is a result of an increased incidence of cardiovascular disease, liver disease and importantly a significant increase in the incidence of serious infections. Of note, HCV infection is also an independent risk factor for graft loss and seems to be associated with greater rates of proteinuria, CAN and TG. It is likely that NODAT and/or HCV-related glomerulonephritis also contributes to the increased prevalence of graft loss reported in this population.

Despite the fact that HCV-infected recipients overall have worse posttransplant outcomes than uninfected patients, they still benefit from transplantation compared to other forms of kidney replacement therapy. In this context, kidney transplantation remains the renal replacement therapy of choice for the HCV-infected ESRD patient. To minimize the adverse consequences of HCV infection after kidney transplantation, several measures are recommended (table 1) including careful management of immunosuppressive therapy and close follow-up of the patient in the posttransplantation period for early detection of proteinuria, allograft dysfunction, infection, NODAT, worsening of liver disease or malignancy.

Table 1. Recommended measures to minimize HCV-related complication after kidney transplantation

HCV-positive patients must be followed carefully to detect deterioration of liver function, infectious diseases, proteinuria, renal dysfunction, NODAT, cardiovascular disease or neoplasia.

Immunosuppression:

- Use a non-aggressive immunosuppressive protocol: no routine use of ATG, ALG or OKT3, except in immunologically high-risk patients.
- Immunosuppression in the maintenance phase depending on the severity of liver disease.
- All immunosuppressive drugs can be used in HCV-positive patients.
- Selected immunosuppressive regimen should be targeted to optimize anti-rejection efficacy, while minimizing the risk of posttransplant diabetes mellitus.

Liver disease:

- At each visit, liver enzymes, bilirubin and prothrombin time should be measured. Antibodies anti-HCV and HCV RNA should be tested at least twice a year.
- Liver biopsy should be considered in patients with abnormal liver function (diagnosis, prognosis, modulation of immunosuppression, possible treatment).
- Extremely important: if HCV-positive patients present severe cholestasis, liver biopsy should be performed immediately. If fibrosing cholestatic hepatitis is present, IFN therapy should be considered on a case-by-case basis.
- In patients with cirrhosis, ultrasonography and α-fetoprotein levels should be monitored frequently to detect hepatocarcinoma early.
- The use of Fibroscan to monitor liver fibrosis could be useful.
- In patients with end-stage liver failure, liver transplantation should be considered.
- Avoid alcohol and potentially hepatotoxic drugs.

Infections:

- Be on the alert for severe infections, such as tuberculosis, and opportunistic infections.
- In case of fever, start effective antibiotic treatment.

HCV-related glomerulonephritis:

- Be on the alert for proteinuria and/or microhematuria.
- In patients with proteinuria/microscopic hematuria, a graft biopsy should be performed.
- In the case of HCV-related glomerulonephritis, antiproteinuric drugs should be started.

HCV-related NODAT:

- Be on the alert for hyperglycemia.
- Patients with hyperglycemia should be referred to a diabetologist.

HCV-related extraliver neoplasia:

- Be on the alert for PTLD.
- Be on the alert for hematological neoplasia.
- Patients with neoplasia should be referred to an oncologist.

References

1 Pereira BJ, Levey AS: Hepatitis C virus infection in dialysis and renal transplantation. Kidney Int 1997;51:981–999.

2 Roth D: Hepatitis C virus: the nephrologist's view. Am J Kidney Dis 1995;25:3–16.

3 Morales JM, Campistol JM: Transplantation in the patient with hepatitis C. J Am Soc Nephrol 2000;11:1343–1353.

4 European Best Practice Guidelines for Renal Transplantation. Section I: Evaluation, selection and preparation of the potential recipient. Nephrol Dial Transplant 2000;15(suppl 7):3–38.

5 KDIGO Clinical Practice Guidelines for the Prevention, Diagnosis, Evaluation, and Treatment of Hepatitis C in Chronic Kidney Disease. Kidney Int 2008;73(suppl 109):S1–S99.

6 Morales JM, Dominguez-Gil B, Sanz-Guajardo D, et al: The influence of hepatitis B and hepatitis C virus infection in the recipient on late renal allograft failure. Nephrol Dial Transplant 2004;19(supply 3):72–76.

7 Burra P, Buda A, Livi U, et al: Occurrence of post-transplant lymphoproliferative disorders among over thousand adult recipients: any role for hepatitis C infection? Eur J Gastroenterol Hepatol 2006;18:1065–1070.

8 Caillard S, Lelong C, Pessione F, Moulin B: Post-transplant lymphoproliferative disorders occurring after renal transplantation in adults: report of 230 cases from the French Registry. Am J Transplant 2006;6:2735–4227.

9 Caillard S, Agodoa LY, Bohen EM, Abbott KC: Myeloma, Hodgkin disease and lymphoid leukaemia after renal transplantation: characteristics, risk factors and prognosis. Transplantation 2006;27:888–895.

10 Corell A, Morales JM, Mandroño A, et al: Immunosuppression induced by hepatitis C virus infection reduces acute renal transplant rejection. Lancet 1995;346:1497–1498.

11 Roth D, Gaynor JJ, Reddy KR, et al: Clinical outcomes in hepatitis C patients before and after kidney transplantation. J Am Soc Nephrol 2011;22:1152–1160.

12 Forman JP, Tolkoff-Rubin N, Pascual M, Lin J: Hepatitis C, acute humoral rejection, and renal allograft survival. J Am Soc Nephrol 2004;15:3249–3255.

13 Morales JM, Marcen R, Andres A, et al: Renal transplantation in patients with hepatitis C virus antibody. A long national experience. NDT Plus 2010;3(suppl 2):ii41–ii46.

14 Moreso F, Ibernon M, Goma M, et al: Subclinical rejection associated with chronic allograft nephropathy in protocol biopsies as a risk factor for late graft loss. Am J Transplant 2006;6:747–752.

15 Rao KV, Ma J: Chronic viral hepatitis enhances the risk of infection but not acute rejection in renal transplant recipients. Transplantation 1996;62:1765–1769.

16 Mitwalli AH, Alam A, Al-Wakeel J, et al: Effect of chronic viral hepatitis on graft survival in Saudi renal transplant patients. Nephron Clin Pract 2006;102:c72–c80.

17 Lopez Medrano F, Fernandez M, Morales JM, et al: Impact of hepatitis C virus infection on the risk of infectious complications after kidney transplantation. Data from the RESITRA/REIPI cohort. Transplantation 2011;92:543–549.

18 Torres J, Aguado JM, San Juan R, et al: Hepatitis C virus, an important risk factor for tuberculosis in immunocompromised: experience with kidney transplantation. Transplant Int 2008;21:873–878.

19 Bloom RD, Sayer G, Fa K, et al: Outcome of hepatitis C virus-infected kidney transplant candidates who remain on the waiting list. Am J Transplant 2005;5:139–144.

20 Abbott KC, Bucci JR, Matsumoto CS, et al: Hepatitis C and renal transplantation in the era of modern immunosuppression. J Am Soc Nephrol 2003;14:2908–2918.

21 Campbell MS, Constantinescu S, Furth EE, Reddy KR, Bloom RD: Effects of hepatitis C-induced liver fibrosis on survival in kidney transplant candidates. Dig Dis Sci 2007;52:2501–2507.

22 Scott DR, Wong JKW, Spicer TS, et al: Adverse impact of hepatitis C virus infection on renal replacement therapy and renal transplant patients in Australia and New Zealand. Transplantation 2010;90:1165–1171.

23 Dominguez-Gil B, Morales JM: Transplantation in the patient with hepatitis C. Transplant Int 2009;22:1117–1131.

24 Legendre C, Garrigue V, Le Bihan C, Mamzer-Bruneel MF, Chaix ML, Landais P, Kreis H, Pol S: Harmful long-term impact of hepatitis C virus infection in kidney transplant recipients. Transplantation 1998;65:667–670.

25 Mathurin P, Mouquet C, Poynard T, et al: Impact of hepatitis B and C virus on kidney transplantation outcome. Hepatology 1999;29:257–263.

26 Maluf DG, Fisher RA, King AL, et al: Hepatitis C virus infection and kidney transplantation: predictors of patient and graft survival. Transplantation 2007;83:853–857.

27 Fabrizi F, Martin P, Dixit V, Bunnapradist S, Dulai G: Hepatitis C virus antibody status and survival after renal transplantation: meta-analysis of observational studies. Am J Transplant 2005;5:1452–1461.

28 Knoll GA, Tankersley MR, Lee JY, et al: The impact of renal transplantation on survival in hepatitis C positive end-stage renal disease patients. Am J Kidney Dis 1997;29:606–614.

29 Pereira BJ, Natov SN, Bouthot, et al: Effects of hepatitis C infection and renal transplantation on survival in end-stage renal disease. The New England Organ Bank Hepatitis C Study Group. Kidney Int 1998;53:1374–1381.

30 Wolfe RA, Ashby VB, Milford El, et al: Comparison of mortality in all patients on dialysis, patients on dialysis awaiting transplantation and recipients of a first cadaveric transplant. N Engl J Med 1999;341:1725–1730.

31 Bruchfeld A, Wilczek H, Einder CG: Hepatitis C infection, time in renal-replacement therapy and outcome after kidney transplantation. Transplantation 2004;78:745–750.

32 Gentil MA, Rocha JL, Rodriguez Algarra G, et al: Impaired kidney transplant survival in patients with antibodies to hepatitis C virus. Nephrol Dial Transplant 1999;94:2455–2460.

33 Mahmoud IM, Elhabasi AF, Elsawy E, at al: The impact of hepatitis C virus viremia on renal graft and patient survival: a 9-year prospective study. Am J Kidney Dis 2004;43:131–139.

34 Lin HH, Huang CC, Huang JY, et al: Impact of HCV infection on first cadaveric renal transplantation, a single center experience. Clin Transplant 2004;18:261–266.

35 Hestin D, Guillemin F, Castin N, et al: Pretransplant hepatitis C virus infection: a predictor of proteinuria after renal transplantation. Transplantation 1998;65:741–744.

36 Cosio FG, Roche Z, Agrawal A, et al: Prevalence of hepatitis C virus in patients with idiopathic glomerulopathies in native and transplanted kidneys. Am J Kidney Dis 1996;28:752–758.

Jose M. Morales, MD
Nephrology Department, Hospital 12 de Octubre
Avenida de Cordoba s/n
ES–28041 Madrid (Spain)
Tel. +34 91 3908619, E-Mail jmorales@h12o.es

Morales JM (ed): Hepatitis C in Renal Disease, Hemodialysis and Transplantation.
Contrib Nephrol. Basel, Karger, 2012, vol 176, pp 87–96

Treatment of Hepatitis C Virus Infection after Kidney Transplantation

Lionel Rostaing[a,c] · Hugo Weclawiak[a] · Jacques Izopet[b,c] · Nassim Kamar[a,c]

[a]Department of Nephrology, Dialysis, and Organ Transplantation, CHU Rangueil, Toulouse University Hospital, [b]Laboratory of Virology, and [c]INSERM U563, IFR 30, Toulouse, France

Abstract

The prevalence of chronic hepatitis C virus (HCV) infection after kidney transplantation (KT) varies a lot from one country to another. In the setting of (powerful) immunosuppression, HCV replication can sharply increase, thereby leading to potential severe HCV-related liver damage such cirrhosis or fibrosing cholestatic hepatitis. In the setting of KT, α-interferon (α-IFN) therapy alone has been associated with a very low sustained virological response (SVR), and a poor tolerance, particularly with regard to the kidney allograft, i.e. it induces acute rejection. The combined use of α-IFN plus ribavirin leads to a greater rate of SVR, but randomized clinical trials are missing in order to evaluate its safety with respect to the allograft function. Ribavirin monotherapy, or ribavirin plus amantadine therapy are not able to induce SVR; ribavirin may have an effect upon HCV-related proteinuria. Finally, it seems advisable to try and eradicate HCV infection prior to KT, i.e. while the patient is on dialysis therapy. After KT, α-IFN plus ribavirin therapy could be attempted only in those patients developing rapid cirrhosis or in those developing fibrosing cholestatic hepatitis or in those having de novo cryoglobulinemic glomerulonephritis within the allograft.

Infection by hepatitis C virus (HCV) leads to chronic liver disease, but also to extrahepatic manifestations. These include mixed cryoglobulinemia, lymphoproliferative disorders and renal disease. HCV infection has been reported to be associated with distinct histological signs of glomerulonephritis in native kidneys. Membranoproliferative glomerulonephritis (MPGN), associated with type II cryoglobulinemia, is the predominant type of HCV-related glomerulonephritis. Less common glomerulonephritis diseases have been reported in HCV-infected patients: these include MPGN without cryoglobulinemia, membranous glomerulonephritis (MGN) [1], focal segmental glomerular sclerosis, proliferative glomerulonephritis, and fibrillary and immunotactoid glomerulopathies. Other anecdotal case reports have also been published: HCV-related IgA nephropathy, rapidly progressive glomerulonephritis, and thrombotic microangiopathy associated with cryoglobulinemic MPGN [1]. However, it is still unknown whether a causative effect between these glomerular diseases and HCV infection exists.

After kidney transplantation (KT), HCV infection can lead to de novo glomerulopathies resulting in impairment of kidney allograft function through various mechanisms. In addition to the HCV-related glomerulopathy described above in native kidneys, acute transplant glomerulopathy, chronic transplant glomerulopathy and renal thrombotic microangiopathy associated with anticardiolipin antibodies, have been described. Thus, in order to avoid recurrence of HCV infection on the kidney allograft, it is advisable to treat with an antiviral therapy HCV+/RNA+ dialysis patients who are candidates for a KT with α-interferon (α-IFN), with or without ribavirin.

In the HCV+ dialysis population, antiviral therapy leads to HCV clearance in ~50% of patients [2]. Moreover, it has been shown that dialysis patients who remain HCV RNA negative before KT have significantly less HCV-related glomerulonephritis after transplantation [3]. In addition, despite heavy immunosuppression, including lymphocyte-depleting agents, these patients have no relapse of HCV infection or occult HCV infection [1]. However, for HCV+/RNA+ patients who undergo KT, HCV infection may have a detrimental effect on patient and allograft survival, and can result in liver dysfunction, such as fibrosing cholestatic hepatitis, as well as cirrhosis, and eventually hepatocarcinoma.

Although many cohort studies show that chronic HCV infection after transplantation is associated with a significant increase in patient death (particularly after 5 years) compared to recipients who are HCV– [5–7], all these studies date back to the 1990s when immunosuppression was different to that used today. It used to rely on azathioprine, cyclosporine, high doses of steroids and sometimes an induction therapy with lymphocyte-depleting agents, all of which can increase HCV replication as compared to HCV RNA concentrations present while patients were on dialysis [8].

A few prospective studies have assessed the liver histology of HCV+/RNA+ KT recipients, though results are controversial. In HCV+patients, Zylberberg et al. [9] showed that liver disease progressed more rapidly in KT recipients comparing to patients with normal renal function or those receiving dialysis. Conversely, we have shown that most HCV+/RNA+ KT patients have almost no progression of HCV-related infection, i.e. changes to their Metavir fibrosis score were similar to those of HCV+/RNA+ dialysis patients, and were significantly lower than those of HCV+/RNA+ patients with normal renal function [10]. These results were sustained after a follow-up of >6 years, during which

KT patients experienced a mean of three posttransplant serial liver biopsies [11]. Nonetheless, some patients (~20%) developed severe liver fibrosis after transplant. Thus, posttransplant antiviral therapy could be considered for these patients, and for those who present with fibrosing cholestatic hepatitis or HCV-related heavy proteinuria [12]. Therapeutic options include α-peg-IFN, ribavirin, and amantadine each alone or as a combined therapy.

Treatments

Anti-HCV Therapy

Anti-HCV therapy may be considered for KT recipients to prevent/reduce HCV-related liver injury. Moreover, because a link has been established between HCV infection and the occurrence of de novo (cryoglobulinemic) MPGN within the kidney allograft, antiviral therapies are an option for HCV+ KT patients presenting with de novo glomerulonephritis to achieve clearance of HCV from the serum and, consequently, to reduce renal injury.

α-Interferon

In studies in the early 1990s, standard α-IFN was given alone and at different doses, i.e. 3–10 million units (MU), three times a week, to small series of KT recipients. Unfortunately, the results were disappointing. It was found that (a) aminotransferase levels improved in only ~50% of cases, (b) virological response while on therapy was only ~25%, (c) sustained virological response (SVR) was very low, and (d) the number of side effects was high, leading to many dropouts [13–15]. One of the major side effects was acute renal failure, which was related to the occurrence of acute-rejection episodes and resulted in some graft losses [15, 16]. It was later shown that most of these rejections were of humoral type [17].

A recent review paper stated that 'posttransplant α-IFN therapy is associated with an increased risk of graft rejection, and given the paucity of information on HCV treatment in solid-organ transplant recipients, there is a great need for large-scale, multi-center randomized controlled trials to determine the optimal approach to HCV infection in this population' [18]. A relatively recent meta-analysis by Fabrizi et al. [19] evaluated the efficacy and safety of antiviral therapy with α-IFN (α-IFN alone or α-IFN plus ribavirin) in renal transplant patients with HCV. They identified 12 clinical trials (102 unique patients), of which only one was a controlled study. The estimated SVR and dropout rates were 18.0% (95% CI, 7.0–29.0) and 35.0% (95% CI, 20–50), respectively. The most frequent side effect that required interruption of treatment was graft dysfunction (n = 28; 71.7%). Meta-regression analyses showed an inverse and significant association between reference year and dropout rate (p = 0.012). They concluded that α-IFN-based therapy for HCV has poor tolerance and safety after RT [19].

Given the above results, it is recommended not to give α-(peg)-IFN alone to HCV+ KT recipients.

α-IFN plus Ribavirin

The efficacy and safety of combined α-IFN plus ribavirin, given to HCV patients on long-term dialysis, was recently evaluated in a meta-analysis of 10 clinical studies (151 unique patients), of which only one (10%) was a controlled clinical trial [2]. Most (97.4%) patients were on long-term hemodialysis. Estimated SVR and dropout rates were 56% (95% CI, 28–84) and 25% (95% CI, 10–40), respectively. The most frequent side effects that required interruption of treatment were anemia (26%) and heart failure (9%). These results occurred irrespective of type of α-IFN (conventional or peg-IFN, peg-IFN-α2a or -α2b), trial design (controlled or cohort study), or clinical characteristics of the patients (naïve, nonresponders or relapsers). The authors' conclusion was that combined antiviral therapy (α-IFN plus ribavirin) gives encouraging results in terms of efficacy and safety among dialysis patients, despite the limited number of patients enrolled in the meta-analysis [2].

What are the data for KT patients? Recently, Pageaux et al. [20] reported on 8 HCV+ renal transplant recipients who began antiviral therapy at a median time of 198.8 months after transplantation. Treatment was scheduled for 24 or 48 weeks according to HCV genotype, i.e. non-1 vs. 1, respectively. α-(peg)-IFN was used at standard doses, i.e. 180 μg/week for peg-IFN-α2a and 1.5 μg/kg/week for peg-IFN-α2b, plus low-dose ribavirin (400 mg/day). Immunosuppression was based on calcineurin inhibitors in 6 cases and on anti-purine agents for the other two; all patients also received low doses of steroids. SVR was observed in 4 of the 8 patients. Three patients with an SVR were genotype 2, one was genotype 1. At baseline, renal dysfunction was moderate in 7 patients and severe in one patient. No patient experienced a rejection episode during or after α-peg-IFN therapy. One patient developed hemolytic uremic syndrome, which eventually resulted in graft loss and a return to dialysis. Pageaux et al. [20] concluded that, for renal transplant recipients treated with α-(peg)-IFN-based therapy, there was a low risk of renal dysfunction, acceptable tolerance and significant virological efficacy.

Sharma et al. [21] gave low-dose α-IFN, i.e. 1.5 MU daily or 3 MU thrice weekly, plus ribavirin, for a period of 2–18 months, to 6 patients. Only 2 patients had an SVR (33.3%), 2 patients relapsed after initial remission, and treatment was stopped for the other 2 patients after 2 months because of graft dysfunction. Overall, 4 patients developed graft dysfunction at some time during α-IFN therapy (66.6%). All patients regained normal creatinine levels after discontinuation of α-IFN, although one patient developed chronic allograft nephropathy, as shown from a kidney biopsy.

Shu et al. [22] reported on 11 renal transplant recipients with active HCV who were treated with ultra-low-dose α-IFN (1 × 10 U, subcutaneously, three times/week) plus ribavirin (600 mg/day) for 48 weeks. Three patients terminated therapy prematurely: one because of acute graft failure and 2 because they developed urosepsis. Only 3 patients had an SVR (27%). Conversely, Schmitz et al. [23] reported on better results; however, this was in the setting of combined liver-kidney transplantation. Hence, in 6 combined liver and kidney transplant recipients who received peg-IFN-α2b (1 μg/kg/weekly) plus ribavirin (600 mg/day) for 48 weeks to treat recurrent HCV, an SVR was achieved in ~50% of patients, and none developed signs of deteriorating kidney function or rejection.

However, overall, these nonrandomized studies had no histological data that compared histology before and after antiviral therapy. In addition, very few patients achieved an SVR in several of these studies, and some patients developed allograft dysfunction.

Ribavirin Monotherapy

Ribavirin (1-β dribofuranosyl-1,2,4-triazole-3-carboxyamide) is a synthetic guanosine analogue that inhibits viral RNA-dependent RNA polymerase by depleting intracellular guanosine pools and interfering with the capping of RNA. Ribavirin monotherapy may decrease HCV-related liver injuries through its immune modulatory properties, even in the absence of an antiviral effect.

The first large study on ribavirin as a monotherapy for HCV+ KT patients was published by Kamar et al. [24]. They evaluated the efficacy and safety of ribavirin as a monotherapy in 16 HCV+ RT patients treated with ribavirin (group A) matched to 32 HCV+ RT patients (group B) who did not receive ribavirin [24]. Ribavirin was started at a daily dose of 1,000 mg, and was then adapted to hemoglobin level. The study was scheduled to last 1 year. They found that ribavirin monotherapy was associated with decreased liver enzyme and serum creatinine levels. When proteinuria was present, it decreased or disappeared. There were no significant changes in HCV viremia. Hemoglobin levels fell dramatically, despite important use of recombinant erythropoietin levels (median, 20,000 IU/week). In 3 cases, ribavirin therapy had to be stopped. In the control group, after 1 year of follow-up, there was a significant increase in serum alanine aminotransferase (ALT) and creatinine values. Proteinuria decreased in only 2 of the 12 patients ($p = 0.03$, compared with group A). In addition, in group A patients they found that liver fibrosis had significantly progressed and there was no improvement in inflammation score [24]. Kamar et al. [25] looked for factors associated with progressive liver fibrosis as being caused by ribavirin-induced hemolysis. Hence, ribavirin induced a significant increase in serum ferritin levels ($p = 0.02$) and intrahepatic iron deposition ($p = 0.04$). Moreover, transferrin level and total iron-binding capacity decreased significantly during ribavirin monotherapy ($p = 0.004$). The side effects of ribavirin may have been due to its accumulation when renal function was impaired, thereby necessitating ribavirin dose adaptations. The authors concluded that 1 year of ribavirin monotherapy seemed to have, at best, no beneficial effect on liver histology, although it improved liver enzyme levels.

In a smaller study, Sharma et al. [21] reported on eight HCV+ KT recipients who were treated with ribavirin alone for a period of 6–24 months, at doses of 400–800 mg daily. As compared to pre-treatment, the mean ALT levels after treatment were significantly reduced (198.4 ± 147.6 and 104.8 ± 66.5 IU/l; $p < 0.05$). ALT levels normalized completely in 3 patients by the end of treatment, improved in 3 patients and deteriorated in 2. HCV-RNA became negative after 6 months of treatment in only one patient. Sharma et al. [21] concluded that ribavirin monotherapy, given to RT recipients with chronic HCV infection, results in a good biochemical response, but is not associated with virological clearance.

Amantadine

Amantadine is an oral antiviral agent that has immunomodulatory effects and has been extensively used to treat influenza. Several studies have reported that oral amantadine can also improve aminotransferase levels in HCV+ patients [26]. It was also suggested that amantadine could potentiate the antiviral effect of a combined regimen of α-IFN plus ribavirin in patients with chronic HCV [27]. However, recent data from HCV+ patients do not demonstrate such a benefit [28].

There are very few data from HCV+ KT patients. Kamar et al. [29] evaluated in an open pilot study the efficacy and safety of amantadine monotherapy in 8 HCV+ RT patients with chronic active hepatitis and increased ALT levels. After 6 months of amantadine therapy (200 mg/day), there was no decrease in HCV viremia (5.87 ± 0.37 log copies/ml at month 6 vs. 5.71 ± 0.5 log copies/ml at baseline; $p > 0.05$). However, they did find a significant decrease in ALT activity (71 ± 17 IU/l at month 6 vs. 100 ± 9 IU/l at baseline; $p = 0.04$), whereas the decrease in aspartate aminotransferase activity did not reach statistical significance. There were no significant changes in liver histology. Clinical and biological tolerance was very good. They concluded that the amantadine monotherapy lacked efficacy in HCV RT patients: it was able to improve liver enzyme levels, but had no impact on either HCV viremia or liver histology.

In a recent prospective randomized controlled study, Calanca et al. [30] evaluated ribavirin therapy alone and amantadine plus ribavirin therapy in HCV+ KT patients. There were three treatments: ribavirin was given at 1,000 mg daily ($n = 7$), or ribavirin was given at 1,000 mg plus amantadine at 200 mg daily ($n = 8$) for 12 months, or no therapy was given (controls, $n = 26$). No significant differences were found between the treatments regarding liver enzyme levels, HCV viremia, liver histology or renal parameters. However, antiviral treatment had to be limited because of anemia, resulting in premature withdrawal of antiviral therapy, and implementation of recombinant erythropoietin (in most patients). The best predictor for tolerability of active treatment was a creatinine clearance rate of >50 ml/min. Calanca et al. [30] concluded that the amantadine plus ribavirin therapy was not superior to the ribavirin monotherapy in RT patients with chronic replicating HCV. However, this result may have been partly because of poor tolerability to both ribavirin and amantadine in patients with impaired renal function, which resulted in several dropouts and, thus, probable subtherapeutic drug dosage.

From the above review of the literature regarding the potential benefit of current antiviral agents to treat HCV RNA+ KT patients, it appears that either a ribavirin monotherapy or ribavirin combined with amantadine are unable to achieve HCV-RNA viral clearance. The use of peg-α-IFN alone is associated with a very low rate of SVR compared to the nonimmunocompromised HCV+ population. Moreover, its use may result in kidney allograft dysfunction, mostly by triggering acute rejection. The combined use of (very low dose) peg-α-IFN plus ribavirin results in a higher sustained virological rate compared to peg-α-IFN alone, although no randomized controlled trials have been conducted on this. Moreover, no follow-up data regarding liver biopsies are available. Thus, it is difficult to conclude with certainty on the potential risk of α-IFN-induced allograft rejection and ribavirin-induced anemia, particularly when estimated glomerular-filtration rate is <50 ml/min.

Therefore, which HCV/RNA+ KT recipients can benefit from anti-HCV therapy after transplantation, i.e. peg-α-IFN plus ribavirin? Recent data show that repeat posttransplant liver biopsies in most HCV-RNA+ KT recipients do not have worsening liver lesions. Roth et al. [31] recently reported on 207 patients who had a liver biopsy before KT. Of these, 44 patients underwent 51 follow-up liver biopsies at ~5-year intervals, either while on a waiting list for a KT or after KT. Advanced fibrosis was present in only 10% of patients biopsied. KT does not seem to accelerate liver injury; 77% of kidney recipients who underwent follow-up biopsies showed stable or improved liver histology. Kamar et al. [11] observed similar findings. They studied 51 anti-HCV+/RNA+ RT patients who underwent liver biopsies every 3–4 years after transplantation (number of liver biopsies: two n = 51; three n = 42; four n = 9). Overall, the progression rate of liver fibrosis was 0.09 ± 0.03 Metavir U/year. They identified three groups of patients: those in whom liver fibrosis remained stable (n = 21), those with progressing liver fibrosis (n = 21) and those with a regression in liver fibrosis (n = 10). In the last two groups, progression and regression of liver fibrosis were gradual during follow-up. Ferritin levels and hepatosiderosis were significantly higher in those with fibrosis. They reported that initial fibrosis stage and high diversification of HVR-1 in the HCV genome, between transplantation and the first liver biopsy, were independent factors associated with regression of liver fibrosis. Kamar et al. [11] concluded that, at >10 years after RT, HCV infection caused harm, as assessed by liver histology, to <50% of patients. Thus, posttransplant sequential liver biopsies may help identify those HCV RNA+ KT patients who develop severe fibrosis, and who could benefit from antiviral therapy. Moreover, HCV RNA+ KT patients who develop a severe life-threatening condition, such as fibrosing cholestatic fibrosis (FCH), could benefit from antiviral therapy, thus, increasing their chances of surviving this severe condition.

Muñoz De Bustillo et al. [32] were the first to describe FCH in HCV+ KT recipients. Of their series of 259 HCV-infected RT patients, 4 (1.5%) presented with FCH. All were receiving steroids, cyclosporine and azathioprine. Shortly after KT (mean: 11.5 months), of these 4, 3 developed hyperbilirubinemia (6.5–mg/dl) and high alkaline phosphatase levels (428–859 IU/l). All 4 subjects developed high γ-glutamyl transpeptidase levels (639–4,270 IU/l), mild aspartate aminotransferase and ALT abnormalities, and high serum HCV RNA. Liver biopsies revealed diffuse fibrosis, leukocyte infiltrates and varying degrees of cholestasis, with typical signs of HCV hepatitis in only one patient. Two patients developed subfulminant liver failure and died at 2 and 3 months after the biopsy. One patient who suffered from hepatic failure received a liver transplant. The fourth patient remained alive on dialysis awaiting a combined kidney and liver transplant.

Delladetsima et al. [33] also reported on a small series of four FCH cases, within a cohort of 73 RT recipients with HCV infection. For these 4 patients, the interval from transplantation to the appearance of liver dysfunction was 1–4 months, and it was 3–11 months until histological diagnosis. The biochemical profile of 3 of these patients was progressive cholestatic syndrome, whereas the 4th patient had only slightly increased ALT and γ-glutamyltransferase levels. Liver histological examination showed a characteristic pattern of FCH in 2 patients, whereas the other 2 patients had changes compatible with early-stage FCH. All patients were anti-HCV negative at the time of transplantation, though 2 patients (one with incomplete and one with complete histological FCH features) seroconverted after 3 and 31 months, respectively. All four patients were HCV-RNA positive at the time of the first liver biopsy and showed high serum HCV RNA levels. HCV genotype was 1b in 3 patients and 3a in one patient. After histological diagnosis, immunosuppression was drastically reduced. Two patients died of sepsis and liver failure at 16 and 18 months after transplantation, whereas the seroconverted patients showed marked improvement in liver disease, which was histologically verified in one patient. Toth et al. [34] have successfully treated 2 similar patients with α-IFN.

It has been shown that cryoglobulinemia is often positive in KT patients, particularly in those who are HCV+. This can result in heavy proteinuria and allograft dysfunction. In this setting, Basse et al. [35] reported on 7 patients, of whom 5 were HCV+, who developed type III cryoglobulinemia-associated MPGN, and had renal function impairment long after transplantation, as well as de novo nephrotic syndrome (n = 5), severe hypertension (n = 5), nephritic syndrome (n = 1) and increased serum creatinine (n = 1). In addition to their baseline standard immunosuppressive medications, the patients were given weekly rituximab infusions: 375 mg/m^2 for 2 weeks in 4 cases, for 3 weeks in one case, and for 4 weeks in 2 cases. This treatment dramatically improved all renal parameters, giving sustained remission of nephrotic syndrome in 3 cases, the disappearance of nephritic syndrome in one patient, and improved nephrotic syndrome in 2 cases, as well as a sustained clearance of cryoglobulins in 6 cases. However, it also resulted in severe infectious complications in 2 cases.

In summary, the data from HCV-related pathologies in KT patients show that it is reasonable to consider antiviral therapy, i.e. peg-α-IFN plus ribavirin in those patients who develop severe liver fibrosis after transplantation or develop fibrosing cholestatic hepatitis. In those who present with cryoglobulinemia-related MPGN, plus heavy proteinuria, rituximab therapy could be attempted. Because of the potential hazard of α-IFN therapy regarding the kidney allograft function, it is advisable to suggest to try and eradicate HCV infection prior to KT to prevent posttransplant HCV-related disorders. In this setting, antiviral therapy is as efficient as in the general population.

References

1 Kamar N, Izopet J, Alric L, Guilbeau-Frugier C, Rostaing L: Hepatitis C virus-related kidney disease: an overview. Clin Nephrol 2008;69:149–160.

2 Fabrizi F, Dixit V, Martin P, Messa P: Combined antiviral therapy of hepatitis C virus in dialysis patients: meta-analysis of clinical trials. J Viral Hepat 2011;18:e263–e269.

3 Cruzado JM, Casanovas-Taltavull T, Torras J, Baliellas C, Gil-Vernet S, Grinyó JM: Pretransplant interferon prevents hepatitis C virus-associated glomerulonephritis in renal allografts by HCV-RNA clearance. Am J Transplant 2003;3:357–360.

4 Kamar N, Toupance O, Buchler M, et al: Evidence that clearance of hepatitis C virus RNA after alpha-interferon therapy in dialysis patients is sustained after renal transplantation. J Am Soc Nephrol 2003;14:2092–2098.

5 Legendre C, Garrigue V, Le Bihan C, et al: Harmful long-term impact of hepatitis C virus infection in kidney transplant recipients. Transplantation 1998;65:667–670.

6 Hanafusa T, Ichikawa Y, Kishikawa H, et al: Retrospective study on the impact of hepatitis C virus infection on kidney transplant patients over 20 years. Transplantation 1998;66:471–476.

7 Mathurin P, Mouquet C, Poynard T, et al: Impact of hepatitis B and C virus on kidney transplantation outcome. Hepatology 1999;29:257.

8 Roth D, Zucker K, Cirocco R, et al: A prospective study of hepatitis C virus infection in renal allograft recipients. Transplantation 1996;61:886.

9 Zylberberg H, Nalpas B, Carnot F, et al: Severe evolution of chronic hepatitis C in renal transplantation: a case control study. Nephrol Dial Transplant 2002;17:129.

10 Alric L, Di-Martino V, Selves J, et al: Long-term impact of renal transplantation on liver fibrosis during hepatitis C virus infection. Gastroenterology 2002;123:1494.

11 Kamar N, Rostaing L, Selves J, et al: Natural history of hepatitis C virus-related liver fibrosis after renal transplantation. Am J Transplant 2005;5:1704.

12 Tang IY, Walzer N, Aggarwal N, et al: Management of the kidney transplant patient with chronic hepatitis C infection. Int J Nephrol 2011;2011:245823.

13 Rostaing L, Izopet J, Baron E, et al: Treatment of chronic hepatitis C with recombinant interferon alpha in kidney transplant recipients. Transplantation 1995;59:1426.

14 Thervet E, Pol S, Legendre C, et al: Low-dose recombinant leukocyte interferon-alpha treatment of hepatitis C viral infection in renal transplant recipients. A pilot study. Transplantation 1994;58:625.
15 Magnone M, Holley JL, Shapiro R, et al: Interferon-alpha-induced acute renal allograft rejection. Transplantation 1995;59:1068.
16 Rostaing L, Modesto A, Baron E, et al: Acute renal failure in kidney transplant patients treated with interferon alpha 2b for chronic hepatitis C. Nephron 1996;74:512.
17 Baid S, Tolkoff-Rubin N, Saidman S, et al: Acute humoral rejection in hepatitis C-infected renal transplant recipients receiving antiviral therapy. Am J Transplant 2003;3:74.
18 Kim E, Ko HH, Yoshida EM: Treatment issues surrounding hepatitis C in renal transplantation: a review. Ann Hepatol 2011;10:5.
19 Fabrizi F, Lunghi G, Dixit V, Martin P: Meta-analysis: anti-viral therapy of hepatitis C virus-related liver disease in renal transplant patients. Aliment Pharmacol Ther 2006;24:1413.
20 Pageaux GP, Hilleret MN, Garrigues V, et al: Pegylated interferon-alpha-based treatment for chronic hepatitis C in renal transplant recipients: an open pilot study. Transpl Int 2009;22:562.
21 Sharma RK, Bansal SB, Gupta A, et al: Chronic hepatitis C virus infection in renal transplant: treatment and outcome. Clin Transplant 2006;20:677.
22 Shu KH, Lan JL, Wu MJ, et al: Ultralow-dose alpha-interferon plus ribavirin for the treatment of active hepatitis C in renal transplant recipients 2004;77:1894.
23 Schmitz V, Kiessling A, Bahra M, et al: Peginterferon alfa-2b plus ribavirin for the treatment of hepatitis C recurrence following combined liver and kidney transplantation. Ann Transplant 2007;12:22.
24 Kamar N, Sandres-Saune K, Selves J, et al: Long-term ribavirin therapy in hepatitis C virus-positive renal transplant patients: effects on renal function and liver histology. Am J Kidney Dis 2003;42:184.
25 Kamar N, Boulestin A, Selves J, et al: Factors accelerating liver fibrosis progression in renal transplant patients receiving ribavirin monotherapy for chronic hepatitis C. J Med Virol 2005;76:61.
26 Smith JP: Treatment of chronic hepatitis C with amantadine. Dig Dis Sci 1997;42:1681.
27 Brillanti S, Foli M, Di Tomaso M, et al: Pilot study of triple antiviral therapy for chronic hepatitis C in interferon alpha non-responders. Ital J Gastroenterol Hepatol 1999;31:130.
28 van Soest H, van der Schaar PJ, Koek GH, et al: No beneficial effects of amantadine in treatment of chronic hepatitis C patients. Dig Liver Dis 2010;42:496.
29 Kamar N, Rostaing L, Sandres-Saune K, et al: Amantadine therapy in renal transplant patients with hepatitis C virus infection. J Clin Virol 2004;30:110.
30 Calanca LN, Fehr T, Jochum W, et al: Combination therapy with ribavirin and amantadine in renal transplant patients with chronic hepatitis C virus infection is not superior to ribavirin alone. J Clin Virol 2007;39:54.
31 Roth D, Gaynor JJ, Reddy KR, et al: Effect of kidney transplantation on outcomes among patients with hepatitis C. J Am Soc Nephrol 2011;22:1152.
32 Muñoz De Bustillo E, Ibarrola C, Colina F, et al: Fibrosing cholestatic hepatitis in hepatitis C virus-infected renal transplant recipients. J Am Soc Nephrol 1998;9:1109.
33 Delladetsima JK, Boletis JN, Makris F, et al: Fibrosing cholestatic hepatitis in renal transplant recipients with hepatitis C virus infection. Liver Transpl Surg 1999;5:294.
34 Toth CM, Pascual M, Chung RT, et al: Hepatitis C virus-associated fibrosing cholestatic hepatitis after renal transplantation: response to interferon-alpha therapy. Transplantation 1998;66:1254.
35 Basse G, Ribes D, Kamar N, et al: Rituximab therapy for mixed cryoglobulinemia in seven renal transplant patients. Transplant Proc 2006;38:2308.

Prof. Lionel Rostaing
Department of Nephrology, Dialysis, and Organ Transplantation Unit, CHU Rangueil
Toulouse University Hospital
1 Avenue J. Poulhès, TSA 50032
FR–31059 Toulouse Cedex 9 (France)
Tel. +33 5 61 32 25 84, E-Mail rostaing.l@chu-toulouse.fr

Morales JM (ed): Hepatitis C in Renal Disease, Hemodialysis and Transplantation.
Contrib Nephrol. Basel, Karger, 2012, vol 176, pp 97–107

Immunosuppression in Hepatitis C Virus-Infected Patients after Kidney Transplantation

Oriol Manuel[a,b] · Seema Baid-Agrawal[d] · Darius Moradpour[a,c] · Manuel Pascual[a]

[a]Transplantation Center, [b]Infectious Diseases Service, and [c]Division of Gastroenterology and Hepatology, University Hospital of Lausanne, Lausanne, Switzerland; [d]Department of Nephrology and Medical Intensive Care, Campus Virchow-Klinikum, Charité Universitätsmedizin Berlin, Berlin, Germany

Abstract

Hepatitis C virus (HCV) infection is an important health problem in kidney transplant recipients with a significantly higher prevalence than in the general population. Kidney transplantation remains the treatment of choice for most HCV-infected patients with end-stage kidney disease, in spite of lower patient and graft survival as compared to HCV-negative patients. Immunosuppression likely has significant consequences on HCV replication and/or disease after transplantation. However, determining the best immunosuppressive strategies after kidney transplantation in the presence of HCV infection remains challenging. The use of induction therapy is not contraindicated, and a short-course induction may actually be beneficial in HCV-infected kidney transplant recipients. Corticosteroid withdrawal may be an acceptable option in HCV-infected patients with specific comorbidities such as diabetes mellitus or osteoporosis. The best calcineurin inhibitor to be used in HCV-infected patients remains to be determined, as there is a lack of large controlled trials addressing this particular issue. Overall, immunosuppressive regimens need to be individualized according to clinical parameters other than HCV, such as the patient's immunological risk and other comorbidities. In conclusion, there is a need for prospective controlled studies to define the optimal immunosuppressive regimen in HCV-infected kidney transplant recipients.

Chronic hepatitis C virus (HCV) infection is a major public health problem, with an estimated prevalence of 2% worldwide [1], the prevalence being significantly higher in kidney transplant recipients [2]. The natural history of chronic

HCV infection in kidney transplant recipients is not completely understood, and the medical management of these patients remains difficult. In 2011, determining the best immunosuppressive strategies after kidney transplantation in the presence of HCV infection remains challenging, as no definite given regimen has proven its clinical superiority. This article will focus on the management of chronic HCV infection in kidney transplant recipients, highlighting the potential impact of the different immunosuppressive drugs on the outcome of HCV infection in this population, as well as discussing some potential areas for future clinical research.

Patient and Graft Survival

In recent years, accumulating evidence has shown kidney transplantation to confer a long-term survival advantage over dialysis in HCV-infected patients and, therefore, it should be considered the treatment of choice for most end-stage renal disease patients with HCV infection [3, 4]. Despite some conflicting reports, however, HCV-infected patients appear to have an overall lower patient and graft survival as compared with HCV-negative transplant recipients. It is postulated that kidney transplantation, with its need for immunosuppression, increases the risk of posttransplant liver disease and new-onset diabetes among HCV-infected patients, which may adversely affect patient survival [2]. HCV infection may also affect graft survival by enhancing the risk of de novo or recurrent glomerulopathies [5, 6].

There have been several publications in the last two decades on the impact of HCV infection on outcomes after kidney transplantation. Studies with short follow-up (<10 years) failed to show significant differences in patient survival between HCV-positive and -negative recipients [7–9]. However, the majority of recent studies, with extended follow-up, show a detrimental effect of HCV infection on patient survival [10–15]. Therefore, the duration of follow-up seems to be crucial in the evaluation of outcomes, as liver disease can develop slowly (or late) after transplantation.

Regarding graft survival, while numerous studies have reported a deleterious effect of HCV [13, 15, 16], an equal number of studies have indicated outcomes that are comparable to those seen in HCV-negative recipients [10–12]. For example, in an observational cohort study, Forman et al. [11] showed that anti-HCV antibody positivity was not significantly associated with death-censored allograft loss, after adjusting for confounding pre- and posttransplant variables. Similarly, Bouthot et al. [10] found no difference in graft survival with 45 months of follow-up. However, in the larger United Network for Organ Sharing (UNOS) study by Meier-Kriesche et al. [13], a trend toward worse death-censored graft survival in HCV-positive patients as early as after 3 years was found. The Australian and New Zealand registry also found a markedly worse graft survival at both 5 and

10 years in HCV-positive recipients [15]. Most frequent causes of graft failure in this study were glomerulonephritis, chronic allograft nephropathy and death in HCV-infected patients. The outcome of HCV-infected kidney recipients is well summarized by a meta-analysis of eight clinical trials including 6,365 patients, which demonstrated a significantly lower patient and graft survival in HCV-infected recipients (adjusted RR 1.79, 95% CI 1.57–2.03, and 1.56, 95% CI 1.35–1.8, respectively) [17]. The increased mortality was partially related to an increase in liver-related mortality. Increased graft loss associated with HCV status has been associated in part with the occurrence of HCV-related renal disease [18].

Apart from differences in study design and follow-up period, severity and duration of HCV infection, liver histology and associated comorbidities at the time of transplantation, differences in immunosuppressive regimens may also be partly responsible for the discordant patient and graft survival outcomes observed in previous studies. The intensity and type of induction and maintenance immunosuppressive regimens may indeed have a significant impact on the course of HCV infection after transplantation.

Impact of Immunosuppression in HCV-Infected Kidney Transplant Recipients

The immunosuppression which needs to be administered after organ transplantation likely has significant consequences on HCV replication and its associated morbidity. The effect of immunosuppression is highlighted by the case of a transplant recipient who had spontaneous resolution of his HCV infection after complete withdrawal of immunosuppression [19]. However, it remains challenging to assess the impact of a specific immunosuppressive drug on the outcome of HCV infection in kidney transplant recipients. First, immunosuppressive drugs are generally given in combination and, frequently, novel strategies of immunosuppression are utilized in clinical studies (e.g. induction with anti-T cell antibodies followed by immunosuppression minimization, etc.). Second, there is a lack of large studies specifically performed in kidney transplant recipients addressing this particular issue. As a result, most of the inference regarding immunosuppression and HCV infection is drawn from studies or reports in liver transplant recipients. Finally, in attempting to determine the most appropriate immunosuppressive regimen after kidney transplantation, the overall risk of other adverse outcomes with each medication, such as the development of acute rejection or posttransplant diabetes mellitus, must be taken into consideration.

Calcineurin Inhibitors

The calcineurin inhibitors (CNI) cyclosporine and tacrolimus remain arguably the most important immunosuppressive drugs used nowadays in the prevention of acute rejection after kidney transplantation. Although the two agents are somewhat similar, there are some differences among them which may be relevant regarding their influence on HCV infection. Tacrolimus is a slightly more potent immunosuppressant than cyclosporine (for a given degree of nephrotoxicity), and it has been associated with lower rates of acute rejection after kidney transplantation [20]. Tacrolimus is currently the preferred CNI in the majority of transplant centers in the US and in many European centers as well. However, in HCV-infected kidney transplant recipients, the use of tacrolimus has been shown to carry a higher risk for posttransplant diabetes mellitus [21]. Interestingly, in vitro studies suggest that cyclosporine may have an inherent anti-HCV activity, inhibiting viral replication, but it is not known whether this may have beneficial clinical implications and possibly protect from the adverse effects of HCV infection after transplantation [22], especially if lower acute rejection rates are observed in patients receiving tacrolimus as compared to cyclosporine. In addition, no significant differences with respect to viral replication and development of liver fibrosis after kidney transplantation have been found in a recent study [23]. In a large study by Luan et al. [24] using data from the Scientific Registry of Transplant Recipients (SRTR) involving more than 75,000 kidney transplant recipients (including 3,708 HCV-infected patients), the use of tacrolimus or cyclosporine was not associated with any survival benefit in HCV-infected patients, i.e. it could not be determined whether one specific CNI has a clear advantage over the other.

Recent literature in liver transplantation by Berenguer et al. [25] and other groups also suggests that overall there are no significant differences between cyclosporine or tacrolimus in posttransplant outcomes in HCV-infected patients. For example, in a meta-analysis of five studies involving 366 patients, patients receiving tacrolimus had similar incidence of graft loss and acute rejection as compared to patients receiving cyclosporine. In a recent study of HCV-positive liver transplant recipients included in the UNOS database, patients receiving cyclosporine were at slightly higher risk for patient death, graft loss and acute rejection as compared to patients receiving tacrolimus [26]. In contrast, in another recent multi-center Spanish cohort study of 410 liver transplant recipients with recurrent hepatitis C treated with pegylated interferon plus ribavirin therapy, cyclosporine was found to be protective against viral relapse, as compared to tacrolimus [27]. Therefore, both after kidney or liver transplantation, the best CNI to be used in HCV-infected patients remains to be determined. However, it appears unlikely that clear differences between the two CNIs will emerge from future clinical studies.

Steroids

Steroids are still widely used in kidney transplantation, at least during the first year after transplant. The possible detrimental relationship between the use of steroids in HCV-infected patients and the outcome of HCV infection has not been clearly established. On the one hand, it has been known for some time that the administration of high-dose or intravenous boluses of steroids for the treatment of rejection is associated with an increased level of replication of HCV [28]. On the other hand, rapid weaning of steroids has been associated with inferior outcomes in HCV-infected liver transplant recipients [29], so that some moderate steroid use might have beneficial effects after transplantation. However, in another study in liver transplant recipients by Humar et al. [30], rapid steroid discontinuation was associated with lower rates of histopathologic hepatitis C recurrence and posttransplant diabetes mellitus. There are scarce data on the influence of steroid use or their withdrawal in kidney transplant recipients with HCV infection. In the study by Luan et al. [24], mortality was not significantly different between patients who received steroids and those who did not (hazard ratio 1.16, $p = 0.44$). In a small clinical study involving 12 HCV-infected kidney transplant recipients, it was found that rapid steroid withdrawal was not associated with a worse outcome [31].

Antimetabolites

Mycophenolate mofetil (MMF) and mycophenolic acid are inhibitors of the metabolism of pyrimidines and have replaced azathioprine in most transplant centers as a standard immunosuppressive drug, in combination with CNI and steroids. Despite being a more potent immunosuppressive drug than azathioprine (as indicated by lower rates of acute rejection in most published studies after organ transplantation), MMF appears to be safe in kidney transplant recipients with chronic HCV infection. In the study by Luan et al. [24], the use of MMF among HCV-infected patients was associated with a 33% lower risk of mortality, suggesting possible beneficial effects of MMF. It should be mentioned that Rostaing et al. [32] found a significant increase of HCV viremia in 14 kidney transplant recipients who received MMF in place of azathioprine (or in addition to a CNI), but it is not clear if this effect had any deleterious consequences because the long-term outcome of these patients was not reported. In a recent study in liver transplant recipients, monotherapy with MMF was associated with better liver fibrosis scores compared to the use of CNI [33], although some reports have described a more severe hepatitis C recurrence in patients receiving MMF [34, 35]. Thus, these conflicting data highlight the difficulty to draw firm conclusions or precise guidelines currently regarding the use of MMF. However, most centers use MMF, in combination with a CNI, for maintenance immunosuppression after transplantation.

mTOR Inhibitors

Because of their potential broad antiviral activity and antiproliferative effects, mTOR inhibitors (sirolimus and everolimus) are two potentially attractive drugs to be included in immunosuppressive protocols for HCV-infected kidney transplant recipients. In an in vitro model of liver fibrosis, sirolimus was associated with reduced fibrogenesis and cell proliferation [36]. There are scarce data, however, on a possible influence of mTOR inhibitors on outcomes of HCV-infected kidney transplant recipients in clinical practice. In the study by Luan et al. [24], the use of mTOR inhibitors in HCV-infected patients was associated with a non-significant 13% higher risk for mortality as compared to patients not receiving mTOR inhibitors. Switch from CNI to sirolimus in a small series of kidney transplant recipients was considered to be safe, but did not result in a significant decrease in HCV viral loads [37]. In liver transplantation, the use of sirolimus was assessed by Asthana et al. [38] in a retrospective study involving 141 liver transplant recipients with HCV-associated cirrhosis. Patients who received sirolimus had lower HCV-associated activity and fibrosis scores on serial liver biopsies. However, there was no difference in the incidence of recurrence of hepatitis or patient survival. Recently, it has been reported that the use of sirolimus was also associated with lower HCV viral load as compared to CNI in liver transplant recipients [39]. One of the problems with the use of mTOR inhibitors is their relatively inferior tolerability as compared to CNI-based regimens, so that at the present time it cannot be recommended to systematically use this class of drugs in HCV-infected kidney transplant recipients.

Induction Therapy

It is still debated whether all induction therapies have a deleterious impact on the outcome of HCV infection after kidney transplantation. The use of OKT3 (a monoclonal depleting antibody against CD3+ cells) has been clearly associated with a higher rate of severe recurrent hepatitis C in liver transplant recipients and, therefore, OKT3 does not appear to be a good choice for induction (or treatment of rejection) in HCV-infected transplant recipients [40]. The relationship between polyclonal T cell-depleting antibodies and HCV infection is more complex. In a retrospective review of 104 HCV-infected kidney transplant recipients, patients who received induction with antithymocyte globulin had similar HCV viral load as compared to patients without induction [41]. Other outcomes were also similar regardless of the induction therapy received. In the study by Luan et al. [24], induction with either depleting or non-depleting antibodies was associated with a 25% lower risk for mortality as compared to patients not receiving induction therapy, possibly due to a lower rejection rate with less anti-rejection therapy needed. In a recent single-center study that evaluated long-term outcome of 110 HCV-infected patients after kidney transplantation utilizing pre- and posttransplant liver biopsies, a subset analysis of 31 recipients showed that patients who received daclizumab had a worse progression of liver fibrosis score than patients receiving antilymphocyte globulins [4].

As for other immunosuppressants, most of the information on the impact of induction therapy on HCV infection comes from studies in liver transplantation. In a randomized controlled clinical trial (n = 64) performed in HCV-infected liver transplant recipients, there were no differences in transaminase levels, HCV viral load, liver fibrosis and inflammation scores in patients receiving either antithymocyte globulin or steroids as induction therapy, suggesting that a short course of antithymocyte globulin induction may not be deleterious [42]. Another randomized controlled trial showed a similar rate of HCV recurrence in recipients receiving daclizumab compared to those receiving thymoglobulin [43]. However, a recent study based on the UNOS database showed that HCV-infected liver transplant recipients who received induction with antithymocyte globulin and steroids had an inferior graft survival than patients receiving daclizumab [44]. This finding, however, was not confirmed in another UNOS analysis, where induction therapy was actually associated with a better patient and graft survival, both in patients receiving either antithymocyte globulin or daclizumab [45]. Overall, although more prospective studies are needed, it may be reasonable to suggest that if induction therapy is administered, a short course would be preferable for HCV-infected patients.

Rituximab

The anti-CD20 monoclonal antibody rituximab is increasingly used in kidney transplantation for the prevention or treatment of humoral rejection and in the treatment of posttransplant lymphoproliferative disorder. Rituximab has also been administered for the treatment of severe HCV-associated mixed cryoglobulinemia in non-transplant patients. Hepatitis flares have been described in HCV-infected patients receiving rituximab for non-Hodgkin lymphoma, indicating than rituximab should be considered with caution in the presence of HCV infection. For example, in a study including 131 HCV-infected patients with diffuse large B-cell lymphoma treated with rituximab, incidence of severe liver toxicity was significantly higher (27%) as compared to non-HCV-infected patients (3%) [46]. In addition, in the subgroup of 34 patients in whom HCV viral load was measured, a significant increase in HCV RNA levels during rituximab therapy compared to baseline was found. After kidney transplantation, some reports have also associated the use of rituximab with a higher incidence of opportunistic infections (mostly bacterial and fungal infections). On the other hand, in a series of 7 HCV-infected kidney transplant recipients, therapy with rituximab was not associated with a flare of chronic hepatitis C, and HCV viral loads remained stable after a 12-month follow-up period [47].

New Compounds

To our knowledge, there is no reported clinical experience regarding the use of the costimulation blocker belatacept in HCV-infected kidney transplant recipients. A related drug, abatacept, was safely used in the non-transplant setting in 2 HCV-infected patients treated for rheumatoid arthritis [48]. Alemtuzumab (Campath) induction was associated with high HCV replication rates in liver transplant recipients in the Pittsburgh experience [49], but data in kidney transplant recipients are lacking, and caution is recommended because this agent can be associated with intense immunosuppression when administered to transplant recipients.

Optimal Immunosuppressive Regimen in HCV-Infected Kidney Transplant Recipients

Determining the most appropriate immunosuppressive regimen for kidney transplant recipients with chronic HCV infection is challenging. The current literature is still somewhat controversial regarding the deleterious (or beneficial) effects of one specific drug on the outcome of HCV infection after transplantation, and therefore, evidence-based guidelines cannot be proposed in 2011. Immunosuppressive regimens need to be individualized according to clinical parameters other than HCV solely, such as the patient's immunological risk and other comorbidities (for example, risk for diabetes mellitus). The use of induction therapy is not contraindicated in these patients and a short-course induction may actually be beneficial in HCV-positive patients via a reduction in the occurrence of acute rejection, thereby avoiding high-dose steroid boluses. No clear advantage appears to exist for the use of anti-IL-2 receptor monoclonal antibodies as compared to antithymocyte globulins. Again, the choice between these drugs should be made taking into account the overall immunological risk of the patient. However, from past experience it can be stated that the OKT3 monoclonal antibody should not be administered in these patients, as it has been associated with severe hepatitis C. Withdrawal of steroids may be an acceptable option in HCV-infected kidney transplant recipients with specific comorbidities such as diabetes mellitus or osteoporosis. However, it is not clear if a low-dose maintenance steroid therapy might have some beneficial effects in the long-term regarding liver disease. MMF and mycophenolic acid appear to be safe in these patients, and should probably be favored over azathioprine. To date, there are insufficient data to recommend the systematic use of mTOR inhibitors in HCV-infected transplant recipients. More debatable is the type of CNI to be used. On the one hand, tacrolimus is associated with a higher risk for the development of posttransplant diabetes mellitus than cyclosporine, whereas, on the other hand, it appears to be associated with better outcomes in terms of acute rejection and possibly allograft survival, even in HCV-infected patients. Clear differences between the two CNIs remain difficult to demonstrate in this patient population.

Conclusions

The immunosuppressive regimen required after organ transplantation is associated with increased HCV replication and, in general, an accelerated and more severe course of HCV-associated liver disease. However, there are no prospective studies directly comparing different immunosuppressive regimens in HCV-infected kidney transplant recipients. Therefore, there is a need to perform prospective controlled studies with long-term follow-up in order to compare different immunosuppressive protocols (e.g. induction vs. no induction, cyclosporine vs. tacrolimus, steroids vs. no steroids, etc.) to more precisely define the optimal immunosuppressive therapy and the consequences of HCV infection after kidney transplantation. The potential beneficial effects of cyclosporine shown in vitro still need to be confirmed in properly designed randomized controlled trials. Given the increasing number of HCV-infected transplant candidates, delineating the optimal immunosuppressive drugs or regimens should be a research priority in kidney transplantation in the upcoming years.

References

1 Shepard CW, Finelli L, Alter MJ: Global epidemiology of hepatitis C virus infection. Lancet Infect Dis 2005;5:558–567.

2 Baid-Agrawal S, Pascual M, Moradpour D, Frei U, Tolkoff-Rubin N: Hepatitis C virus infection in haemodialysis and kidney transplant patients. Rev Med Virol 2008;18:97–115.

3 Bloom RD, Sayer G, Fa K, Constantinescu S, Abt P, Reddy KR: Outcome of hepatitis C virus-infected kidney transplant candidates who remain on the waiting list. Am J Transplant 2005;5:139–144.

4 Roth D, Gaynor JJ, Reddy KR, et al: Effect of kidney transplantation on outcomes among patients with hepatitis C. J Am Soc Nephrol 2011;22:1152–1160.

5 Baid-Agrawal S, Farris AB, Pascual M, et al: Overlapping pathways to transplant glomerulopathy: chronic humoral rejection, hepatitis C infection and thrombotic microangiopathy. Kidney Int 2011, Epub ahead of print.

6 Baid S, Cosimi AB, Tolkoff-Rubin N, Colvin RB, Williams WW, Pascual M: Renal disease associated with hepatitis C infection after kidney and liver transplantation. Transplantation 2000;70:255–261.

7 Genesca J, Vila J, Cordoba J, et al: Hepatitis C virus infection in renal transplant recipients: epidemiology, clinical impact, serological confirmation and viral replication. J Hepatol 1995;22:272–277.

8 Kliem V, van den Hoff U, Brunkhorst R, et al: The long-term course of hepatitis C after kidney transplantation. Transplantation 1996;62:1417–1421.

9 Roth D, Zucker K, Cirocco R, et al: A prospective study of hepatitis C virus infection in renal allograft recipients. Transplantation 1996;61:886–889.

10 Bouthot BA, Murthy BV, Schmid CH, Levey AS, Pereira BJ: Long-term follow-up of hepatitis C virus infection among organ transplant recipients: implications for policies on organ procurement. Transplantation 1997;63:849–853.

11 Forman JP, Tolkoff-Rubin N, Pascual M, Lin J: Hepatitis C, acute humoral rejection, and renal allograft survival. J Am Soc Nephrol 2004;15:3249–3255.

12 Mathurin P, Mouquet C, Poynard T, et al: Impact of hepatitis B and C virus on kidney transplantation outcome. Hepatology 1999;29:257–263.

13 Meier-Kriesche HU, Ojo AO, Hanson JA, Kaplan B: Hepatitis C antibody status and outcomes in renal transplant recipients. Transplantation 2001;72:241–244.

14 Morales JM, Dominguez-Gil B, Sanz-Guajardo D, Fernandez J, Escuin F: The influence of hepatitis B and hepatitis C virus infection in the recipient on late renal allograft failure. Nephrol Dial Transplant 2004;19(suppl 3):iii72–iii76.

15 Scott DR, Wong JK, Spicer TS, et al: Adverse impact of hepatitis C virus infection on renal replacement therapy and renal transplant patients in Australia and New Zealand. Transplantation 2010;90:1165–1171.
16 Legendre C, Garrigue V, Le BC, et al: Harmful long-term impact of hepatitis C virus infection in kidney transplant recipients. Transplantation 1998;65:667–670.
17 Fabrizi F, Martin P, Dixit V, Bunnapradist S, Dulai G: Hepatitis C virus antibody status and survival after renal transplantation: meta-analysis of observational studies. Am J Transplant 2005;5:1452–1461.
18 Cruzado JM, Carrera M, Torras J, Grinyo JM: Hepatitis C virus infection and de novo glomerular lesions in renal allografts. Am J Transplant 2001;1:171–178.
19 Somsouk M, Lauer GM, Casson D, et al: Spontaneous resolution of chronic hepatitis C virus disease after withdrawal of immunosuppression. Gastroenterology 2003;124:1946–1949.
20 Webster AC, Woodroffe RC, Taylor RS, Chapman JR, Craig JC: Tacrolimus versus ciclosporin as primary immunosuppression for kidney transplant recipients: meta-analysis and meta-regression of randomised trial data. BMJ 2005;331:810.
21 Baid S, Tolkoff-Rubin N, Farrell ML, et al: Tacrolimus-associated posttransplant diabetes mellitus in renal transplant recipients: role of hepatitis C infection. Transplant Proc 2002;34:1771–1773.
22 Watashi K, Hijikata M, Hosaka M, Yamaji M, Shimotohno K: Cyclosporin A suppresses replication of hepatitis C virus genome in cultured hepatocytes. Hepatology 2003;38:1282–1288.
23 Kahraman A, Witzke O, Scherag A, et al: Impact of immunosuppressive therapy on hepatitis C infection after renal transplantation. Clin Nephrol 2011;75:16–25.
24 Luan FL, Schaubel DE, Zhang H, et al: Impact of immunosuppressive regimen on survival of kidney transplant recipients with hepatitis C. Transplantation 2008;85:1601–1606.
25 Berenguer M, Royuela A, Zamora J: Immunosuppression with calcineurin inhibitors with respect to the outcome of HCV recurrence after liver transplantation: results of a meta-analysis. Liver Transpl 2007;13:21–29.
26 Irish W, Arcona S, Bowers D, Trotter JF: Cyclosporine versus tacrolimus treated liver transplant recipients with chronic hepatitis C: outcomes analysis of the UNOS/OPTN Database. Am J Transplant 2011;11:1676–1685.
27 ReViS-TC Study Group: Cyclosporine a-based immunosuppression reduces relapse rate after antiviral therapy in transplanted patients with hepatitis C virus infection: a large multicenter cohort study. Transplantation 2011;92:334–340.
28 Berenguer M, Prieto M, Cordoba J, et al: Early development of chronic active hepatitis in recurrent hepatitis C virus infection after liver transplantation: association with treatment of rejection. J Hepatol 1998;28:756–763.
29 Berenguer M, Aguilera V, Prieto M, et al: Significant improvement in the outcome of HCV-infected transplant recipients by avoiding rapid steroid tapering and potent induction immunosuppression. J Hepatol 2006;44:717–722.
30 Humar A, Crotteau S, Gruessner A, et al: Steroid minimization in liver transplant recipients: impact on hepatitis C recurrence and post-transplant diabetes. Clin Transplant 2007;21:526–531.
31 Akalin E, Murphy B, Sehgal V, Ames S, Daly L, Bromberg JS: Rapid steroid withdrawal in hepatitis C virus-positive kidney transplant recipients. Clin Transplant 2004;18:384–389.
32 Rostaing L, Izopet J, Sandres K, Cisterne JM, Puel J, Durand D: Changes in hepatitis C virus RNA viremia concentrations in long-term renal transplant patients after introduction of mycophenolate mofetil. Transplantation 2000;69:991–994.
33 Manzia TM, Angelico R, Toti L, et al: Long-term, maintenance MMF monotherapy improves the fibrosis progression in liver transplant recipients with recurrent hepatitis C. Transpl Int 2011;24:461–468.

34 Berenguer M, Crippin J, Gish R, et al: A model to predict severe HCV-related disease following liver transplantation. Hepatology 2003;38:34–41.
35 Burak KW, Kremers WK, Batts KP, et al: Impact of cytomegalovirus infection, year of transplantation, and donor age on outcomes after liver transplantation for hepatitis C. Liver Transpl 2002;8:362–369.
36 Zhu J, Wu J, Frizell E, et al: Rapamycin inhibits hepatic stellate cell proliferation in vitro and limits fibrogenesis in an in vivo model of liver fibrosis. Gastroenterology 1999;117:1198–1204.
37 Gallego R, Henriquez F, Oliva E, et al: Switching to sirolimus in renal transplant recipients with hepatitis C virus: a safe option. Transplant Proc 2009;41:2334–2336.
38 Asthana S, Toso C, Meeberg G, et al: The impact of sirolimus on hepatitis C recurrence after liver transplantation. Can J Gastroenterol 2011;25:28–34.
39 Wagner D, Kniepeiss D, Schaffellner S, et al: Sirolimus has a potential to influent viral recurrence in HCV positive liver transplant candidates. Int Immunopharmacol 2010;10:990–993.
40 Rosen HR, Shackleton CR, Higa L, et al: Use of OKT3 is associated with early and severe recurrence of hepatitis C after liver transplantation. Am J Gastroenterol 1997;92:1453–1457.
41 Rodrigues A, Pinho L, Lobato L, et al: Hepatitis C virus genotypes and the influence of the induction of immunosuppression with anti-thymocyte globulin (ATG) on chronic hepatitis in renal graft recipients. Transpl Int 1998;11(suppl 1):S115–S118.
42 Nair S, Loss GE, Cohen AJ, Eason JD: Induction with rabbit antithymocyte globulin versus induction with corticosteroids in liver transplantation: impact on recurrent hepatitis C virus infection. Transplantation 2006;81:620–622.
43 Kamar N, Borde JS, Sandres-Saune K, et al: Induction therapy with either anti-CD25 monoclonal antibodies or rabbit antithymocyte globulins in liver transplantation for hepatitis C. Clin Transplant 2005;19:83–89.
44 Uemura T, Schaefer E, Hollenbeak CS, Khan A, Kadry Z: Outcome of induction immunosuppression for liver transplantation comparing anti-thymocyte globulin, daclizumab, and corticosteroid. Transpl Int 2011;24:640–650.
45 Moonka DK, Kim D, Kapke A, Brown KA, Yoshida A: The influence of induction therapy on graft and patient survival in patients with and without hepatitis C after liver transplantation. Am J Transplant 2010;10:590–601.
46 Ennishi D, Maeda Y, Niitsu N, et al: Hepatic toxicity and prognosis in hepatitis C virus-infected patients with diffuse large B-cell lymphoma treated with rituximab-containing chemotherapy regimens: a Japanese multicenter analysis. Blood 2010;116:5119–5125.
47 Kamar N, Sandres-Saune K, Rostaing L: Influence of rituximab therapy on hepatitis C virus RNA concentration in kidney-transplant patients. Am J Transplant 2007;7:2440.
48 Mahajan TD, Hooker R, Maher L, Brown G, Reimold A: Abatacept therapy for rheumatoid arthritis in the setting of hepatitis C infection. J Clin Rheumatol 2010;16:332–334.
49 Marcos A, Eghtesad B, Fung JJ, et al: Use of alemtuzumab and tacrolimus monotherapy for cadaveric liver transplantation: with particular reference to hepatitis C virus. Transplantation 2004;78:966–971.

Manuel Pascual, MD
Transplantation Center, BH 10 226, University Hospital of Lausanne (CHUV)
CH–1011 Lausanne (Switzerland)
Tel. +41 21 314 2403, E-Mail Manuel.Pascual@chuv.ch

Morales JM (ed): Hepatitis C in Renal Disease, Hemodialysis and Transplantation.
Contrib Nephrol. Basel, Karger, 2012, vol 176, pp 108–116

Impact of Extrahepatic Complications (Diabetes and Glomerulonephritis) Associated with Hepatitis C Virus Infection after Renal Transplantation

Josep M. Cruzado · Oriol Bestard · Josep M. Grinyó

Nephrology Department, Hospital Universitary de Bellvitge, University of Barcelona, IDIBELL, L'Hospitalet de Llobregat, Barcelona, Spain

Abstract

Hepatitis C virus (HCV) infection is associated with some extrahepatic complications, like diabetes, cryoglobulinemia, and membranoproliferative glomerulonephritis. Each of these complications has important implications in the renal allograft recipient. Hence, HCV infection is strongly associated with a lower patient and graft survival in renal transplantation. The increased risk of death in HCV-infected renal allograft recipients has been attributed to cardiovascular mortality, linked someway to the insulin resistance and high risk of new-onset diabetes, rather than to the progression of HCV-related liver disease. On the other hand, graft survival is hampered by the occurrence of de novo HCV-related glomerulonephritis and the higher risk of chronic humoral rejection in this population.

Chronic hepatitis C affects approximately 170 million people worldwide [1]. Hepatitis C virus (HCV) infection leads to cirrhosis and liver cancer, and is the main indication for liver transplantation [2]. HCV infection is further associated with some extrahepatic complications, like diabetes, cryoglobulinemia, and membranoproliferative glomerulonephritis (MPGN). Each of these complications has important implications in the renal allograft recipient [1].

HCV infection prevalence in kidney transplantation is rather variable depending on geographical areas. HCV incidence has been progressively reduced in some European countries due to the implementation of very active policies for avoiding transmission into dialysis units as well as performing HCV treatment before transplantation. However, in many countries it remains a major health problem, with HCV prevalence in the renal transplant population as high as 40% [3].

HCV infection is strongly associated with lower patient and graft survival in renal transplantation [4]. The increased risk of death in HCV-infected renal allograft recipients has been attributed to cardiovascular mortality [5], linked someway to insulin resistance and high risk of new-onset diabetes (NODAT) [6], rather than to the progression of HCV-related liver disease [7]. On the other hand, graft survival is hampered by the presence of HCV-related glomerulonephritis [8] and the higher risk of chronic humoral rejection among this population [9].

HCV Infection as Risk Factor for New-Onset Diabetes after Transplantation

In renal transplantation, NODAT incidence is quite variable depending on its definition, ranging from 2 to 53% [10]. An association between HCV and the occurrence of NODAT has been observed in both liver and kidney transplant recipients, as well as in general population. Actually, HCV prevalence in diabetics is 2.5 times higher than in non-diabetics [1]. Although cirrhosis is known to be associated with acquired abnormalities in glucose metabolism, HCV by itself, independent of the severity of the liver disease is a risk factor for diabetes.

Abnormalities in glucose metabolism in HCV-infected patients are mainly related to insulin resistance, although impaired liver glucose uptake, hepatic glycogenesis inhibition as well as a direct cytopathic effect of HCV on pancreatic beta cells have also been described [1, 10]. Insulin resistance noted in the setting of HCV infection appears to be multifactorial and it is mediated, at least in part, by some proinflammatory cytokines, such as tumor necrosis factor-α and interleukin-6 [11].

A systematic review performed in HCV-positive renal transplant patients reported an odds ratio for NODAT of 3.97 with a 95% confidence interval of 1.83 to 8.61, thus providing a link between HCV, diabetes and cardiovascular disease [12]. The relationship between HCV and NODAT after transplantation is influenced by the presence of traditional risk factors such as obesity, older age, ethnicity (especially African-American and Hispanic) and metabolic syndrome. Furthermore, in the renal transplant setting, there are additional risk factors for diabetes that become synergic with those classical and those specifically related to HCV infection. Gathering all risk factors explains the high incidence of NODAT among HCV-infected transplant recipients [13].

Immunosuppression is definitely one of such risk factors related to transplantation [10]. Actually, in HCV renal transplant recipients NODAT appears within the first months after transplantation when the higher doses of immunosuppression are given. Whether this effect is directly related to immunosuppression or indirectly related to the enhanced HCV replication induced by immunosuppression has not been completely elucidated. Nevertheless, the fact that NODAT was more strongly related to donor rather than recipient HCV seropositivity suggests that acute peritransplant infection is a major player accounting for diabetes [10]. On the other hand, some immunosuppressive drugs are intrinsically risk factors for diabetes, in particular corticosteroids and calcineurin inhibitors (CNIs). Steroid avoidance or discontinuation is recommended whenever possible, although there are no definitive data supporting its beneficial effect in this setting [3, 10]. Regarding CNIs, there is strong evidence supporting that tacrolimus rather than cyclosporine is a major risk factor for NODAT in HCV-infected renal allograft recipients [14].

HCV-Related Glomerulonephritis in Renal Allografts

HCV infection is a major risk factor for renal allograft loss [15]. This effect is so strong that HCV remains as independent predictor of graft outcome even in protocol biopsy studies [16]. Some authors suggest that the deleterious impact of HCV on graft survival is not completely derived by the viral infection but mediated by the high immunological risk showed by HCV-infected population [9]. In fact, HCV-infected patients are frequently retransplants with more prolonged time of renal disease, and eventually have enhanced cellular and humoral immune responses. Cosio et al. [17] some years ago described HCV infection as a risk factor for glomerulitis and transplant glomerulopathy; both entities are currently associated with the presence of anti-HLA antibodies and antibody-mediated rejection.

Although all these caveats regarding the confounding effects of the humoral immune response on HCV-related renal pathology could apply in some cases, it is also true that HCV infection is certainly related to autoimmunity and glomerular disease [18–21]. For instance, the same group arguing for the role of humoral immunity described the association between HCV infection and thrombotic microangiopathy in renal allografts due to the presence of pretransplant anticardiolipin antibodies [22]. Although interesting and previously described in association with HCV infection, this entity is seldom encountered in HCV transplant recipients.

HCV-infected renal as well as liver allograft recipients are prone to developing immune complex-mediated glomerulonephritis as it happens in nontransplanted patients [23, 24]. Some indirect data support this effect. Hestin et al. [25] identified HCV infection as a major risk for developing posttransplant proteinuria. In 1995, Roth et al. [23] reported for the first time de novo MPGN in HCV-infected renal allograft recipients. These authors were not able to demonstrate cryoglobulinemia in these patients although they found some indirect data already suggesting presence of circulating immune complexes. Then, Cruzado et al. [26] described presence of HCV-related type II mixed cryoglobulinemia (IgM-κ monoclonal) in those patients with de novo GNMP after transplantation. In contrast to HCV-related MPGN in non-transplanted patients, HCV-infected allografts show very low cryocrit levels, usually below 5%. This fact may provide explanation for limitations in detection as well as characterization of cryoglobulins among this population. Furthermore, HCV-RNA is usually much higher in cryocrit than in serum, suggesting that HCV has a pathogenic role in the cryoglobulinemia. Accordingly, these patients may have classical complement pathway activation. Clinical manifestations of HCV-related MPGN are hypertension, microhematuria, proteinuria and renal dysfunction, sometimes associated with nephrotic syndrome. Renal biopsy shows variable degree of chronic damage in all compartments associated with focal or diffuse mesangial proliferation, double contours and parietal IgM and C3 deposits by immunofluorescence (fig. 1). However, sometimes pathological diagnosis is difficult, and electron microscopy examination becomes necessary in order to differentiate MPGM from transplant glomerulopathy. In the case of MPGN, there are subendothelial electron-dense deposits, whereas in transplant glomerulopathy there is radiolucent areas in the glomerular baseline membrane. In some cases of MPGN and transplant glomerulopathy, coexistence has been described [27], thus supporting the role of both humoral immunity and autoimmunity as harmful partners accounting for the worse outcome of HCV renal allografts. Morales et al. [28] described membranous glomerulonephritis (MGN) associated with HCV in renal allografts. MGN is the most frequent type of de novo glomerulonephritis in HCV-negative renal allografts. Nephrotic syndrome is usually present. There is no clear pathogenic mechanism connecting HCV with MGN since cryoglobulins or immune complexes as well as complement activation are usually absent.

Prevalence of glomerular lesions in HCV renal allografts varies depending on analyzing protocol or biopsies for cause. Moreover, sometimes the pathological diagnosis is quite difficult to carry out due to presence of mild abnormalities and the overlapping immunological damage. Nevertheless, estimated prevalence is 5–15% [3]. In a study performed in our centre [15] on biopsies for cause, the most frequent glomerulonephritis associated with HCV infection was MPGN followed by MGN. The diagnosis of de novo glomerulonephritis in this population is clinically relevant since it is associated with an accelerated loss of the graft. Even those patients who have lost a previous graft due to de novo HCV-related glomerulonephritis, display an early and more aggressive form of the disease in subsequent transplants.

There is no definitive explanation accounting for the special susceptibility of the renal allograft for developing MPGN. Immunosuppression may be the cause of the very low levels of circulating cryoglobulins observed after transplantation.

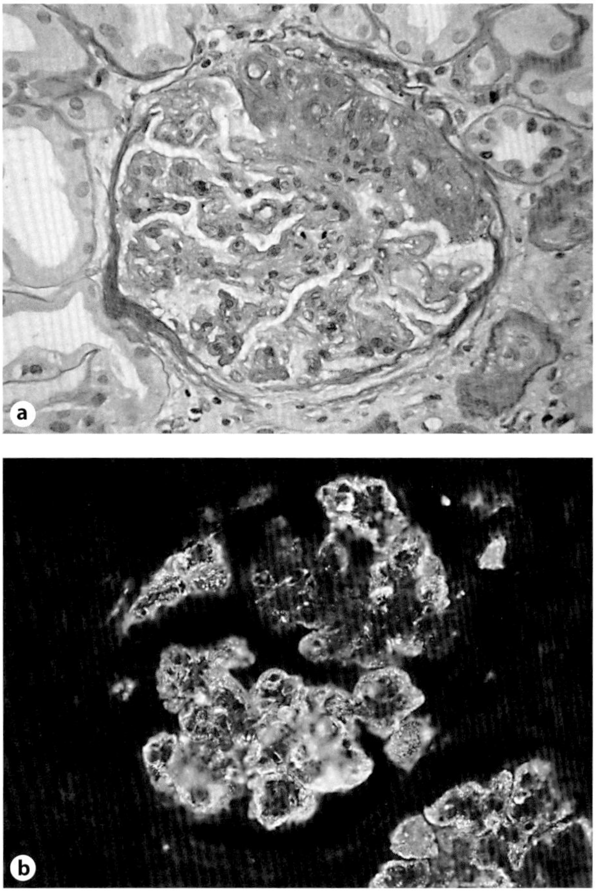

Fig. 1. Histological features of HCV-related de novo MPGN after renal transplantation. Light microscopy and immunofluorescence. **a** Lobular accentuation, mesangial expansion, focal and segmental mesangial hypercellularity and double contour images on some peripheral loops. PAS stain. ×400. **b** Irregular parietal and paramesangial IgM deposits.

However, MPGN is developed despite these low levels of circulating immune complexes. Theoretically, the renal allograft could express more proinflammatory cytokines than the native kidney. Inflammation may increase renal expression of Toll-like receptor 3 (TLR3), in particular in mesangial cells [29, 30]. HCV double-strand RNA could bind to TLR3, therefore producing amplification of the inflammatory response and finally MPGN (fig. 2).

Unfortunately, treatment of de novo HCV-related glomerulonephritis is mainly symptomatic [31, 32]. There is no evidence regarding any specific immunosuppressant acting neither as a risk nor protective factor in this setting. Although there are positive experiences regarding interferon treatment in HCV recurrence after liver transplantation [33], the majority of clinicians

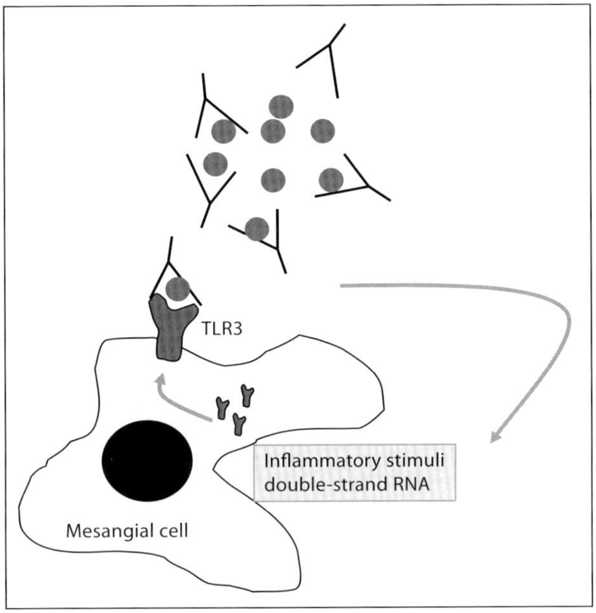

Fig. 2. Innate immunity and HCV-associated glomerulonephritis. Under certain inflammatory stimuli, mesangial cells could express TLR3. Immune complexes containing HCV may bind to TLR3 on mesangial cells, inducing local production of some chemokines and cytokines, which may promote mononuclear cell recruitment and mesangial apoptosis.

agree that interferon should not be administered in renal allograft recipients due to the associated risk of acute rejection and graft loss [34, 35]. There are also some positive experiences with the use of ribavirine [36], although this treatment can induce hemolytic anemia in cases of renal insufficiency, and in monotherapy it is unable to induce sustained viral response. More recently, some authors reported success using rituximab in cases of HCV-related MPGN [37–39]. In our experience [40], rituximab treatment was associated with disappearance of cryoglobulinemia and the glomerular subendothelial immune deposits. However, rituximab treatment may induce overimmunosuppression and may increase viral replication. New antiviral drugs may be available soon in order to overcome limitation of current HCV treatments. Therefore, recommendations regarding HCV and renal transplantation are based on prevention rather than treatment of HCV-related glomerulonephritis [3]. In fact, treatment of HCV-infected renal transplant candidates either by interferon or interferon plus ribavirine can induce sustained viral response in at least 50% of patients [41]. The HCV viral response is usually maintained after transplantation and more importantly, as demonstrated by our group, HCV clearance before transplantation avoids development of HCV-related glomerular lesions after transplantation [42].

Acknowledgments

This research was supported by The Red de Investigación Renal (REDinREN, ISCIII 06/0016).

References

1 Sabharwal S, Delgado-Borrego A, Chung RT: Extrahepatic hepatitis C virus after transplantation: diabetes and renal dysfunction. Liver Transpl 2008;14(suppl 2):S51–S57.
2 Alter MJ, Margolis HS, Krawczynski K, Judson FN, Mares A, Alexander WJ, et al: The natural history of community acquired hepatitis C in the United States. The Sentinel Counties Chronic Non-A, Non-B Hepatitis Study Team. N Engl J Med 1992;327:1899–1905.
3 Perico N, Cattaneo D, Bikbov B, Remuzzi G: Hepatitis C infection and chronic renal diseases. Clin J Am Soc Nephrol 2009;4:207–220.
4 Huskey J, Wiseman AC: Chronic viral hepatitis in kidney transplantation. Nat Rev Nephrol 2011;7:156–165.
5 Abbott KC, Lentine KL, Bucci JR, Agodoa LY, Koff JM, Holtzmuller KC, Schnitzler MA: Impact of diabetes and hepatitis after kidney transplantation on patients who are affected by hepatitis C virus. J Am Soc Nephrol 2004;15:3166–3174.
6 Roth D, Gaynor JJ, Reddy KR, Ciancio G, Sageshima J, Kupin W, Guerra G, Chen L, Burke GW 3rd: Effect of kidney transplantation on outcomes among patients with hepatitis C. J Am Soc Nephrol 2011;22:1152–1160.
7 Bestard O, Cruzado JM, Torras J, Gil-Vernet S, Serón D, Moreso F, Rama I, Grinyó JM: Long-term effect of hepatitis C virus chronic infection on patient and renal graft survival. Transplant Proc 2005;37:3774–3777.
8 Cruzado JM, Torras J, Gil-Vernet S, Grinyó JM: Glomerulonephritis associated with hepatitis C virus infection alter renal transplantation. Nephrol Dial Transplant 2000;15(suppl 8):65–67.
9 Forman JP, Tolkoff-Rubin N, Pascual M, Lin J: Hepatitis C, acute humoral rejection, and renal allograft survival. J Am Soc Nephrol 2004;15:3249–3255.
10 Bloom RD, Lake JR: Emerging issues in hepatitis C virus-positive liver and kidney transplant recipients. Am J Transplant 2006;6:2232–2237.
11 Shintani Y, Fujie H, Miyoshi H, Tsutsumi T, Tsukamoto K, Kimura S, Moriya K, Koike K: Hepatitis C virus infection and diabetes: direct involvement of the virus in the development of insulin resistance. Gastroenterology 2004;126:840–848.
12 Fabrizi F, Martin P, Dixit V, Bunnapradist S, Kanwal F, Dulai G: Post-transplant diabetes mellitus and HCV seropositive status after renal transplantation: meta-analysis of clinical studies. Am J Transplant 2005;5:2433–2440.
13 Räkel A, Karelis AD: New-onset diabetes after transplantation: risk factors and clinical impact. Diabetes Metab 2011;37:1–14.
14 Bloom RD, Rao V, Weng F, Grossman RA, Cohen D, Mange KC: Association of hepatitis C with posttransplant diabetes in renal transplant patients on tacrolimus. J Am Soc Nephrol 2002;13:1374–1380.
15 Cruzado JM, Carrera M, Torras J, Grinyó JM: Hepatitis C virus infection and de novo glomerular lesions in renal allografts. Am J Transplant 2001;1:171–178.
16 Moreso F, Ibernon M, Gomá M, et al: Subclinical rejection associated with chronic allograft nephropathy in protocol biopsies as a risk factor for late graft loss. Am J Transplant 2006;6:747–752.
17 Cosio FG, Sedmak DD, Henry ML, Al Haddad C, Falkenhain ME, Elkhammas EA, Davies EA, Bumgardner GL, Ferguson RM: The high prevalence of severe early posttransplant renal allograft pathology in hepatitis C positive recipients. Transplantation 1996;62:1054–1059.
18 Agnello V, Chung RT, Kaplan LM: A role for hepatitis C virus infection in type II cryoglobulinemia. N Engl J Med 1992;327:1490–1495.

19 Agnello V, De Rosa F: Extrahepatic disease manifestations of HCV infection: some current issues. J Hepatol 2004;40:341–352.
20 D'Amico G, Fornasieri A: Cryoglobulinemic glomerulonephritis: a membranoproliferative glomerulonephritis induced by hepatitis C virus. Am J Kidney Dis 1995;25:361–369.
21 Johnson RJ, Gretch Dr, Yamabe H, et al: Membranoproliferative glomerulonephritis associated with hepatitis C virus infection. N Engl J Med 1993;328:465–470.
22 Baid S, Pascual M, Williams WW Jr, Tolkoff-Rubin N, Johnson SM, Collins B, Chung RT, Delmonico FL, Cosimi AB, Colvin RB: Renal thrombotic microangiopathy associated with anticardiolipin antibodies in hepatitis C-positive renal allograft recipients. J Am Soc Nephrol 1999;10:146–153.
23 Roth D, Cirocco R, Zucker K, et al: De novo membranoproliferative glomerulonephritis in hepatitis C virus-infected renal allograft recipients. Transplantation 1995;59:1676–1682.
24 Cantarell MC, Charco R, Capdevila L, et al: Outcome of hepatitis C virus-associated membranoproliferative glomerulonephritis after liver transplantation. Transplantation 1999;68:1131–1134.
25 Hestin D, Guillemin F, Castin N, et al: Pretransplant hepatitis C virus infection: a predictor of proteinuria after renal transplantation. Transplantation 1998;65:741–744.
26 Cruzado JM, Gil-Vernet S, Ercilla G, et al: Hepatitis C virus-associated membranoproliferative glomerulonephritis in renal allografts. J Am Soc Nephrol 1996;7:2469–2475.
27 Gallay BJ, Alpers CE, Davis CL, Schultz MF, Johnson RJ. Glomerulonephritis in renal allografts associated with hepatitis C infection: a possible relationship with transplant glomerulopathy in two cases. Am J Kidney Dis 1995;26:662–667
28 Morales JM, Pascual-Capdevila J, Campistol JM, Fernandez-Zatarain G, Muñoz MA, Andres A, Praga M, Martinez MA, Usera G, Fuertes A, Oppenheimer F, Artal P, Darnell A, Rodicio JL: Membranous glomerulonephritis associated with hepatitis C virus infection in renal transplant patients. Transplantation 1997;63:1634–1639.
29 Wörnle M, Schmid H, Banas B, et al: Novel role of toll-like receptor 3 in hepatitis C-associated glomerulonephritis. Am J Pathol 2006;168:370–385.
30 Sansonno D, Lauletta G, Montrone M, Grandaliano G, Schena FP, Dammacco F: Hepatitis C virus RNA and core protein in kidney glomerular and tubular structures isolated with laser capture microdissection. Clin Exp Immunol 2005;140:498–506.
31 Natov SN, Pereira BJG: Management of hepatitis C infection in renal transplant recipients. Am J Transplant 2002;2:483–490.
32 Morales JM, Campistol JM: Disease of the month: transplantation in the patient with hepatitis C. J Am Soc Nephrol 2000;11:1343–1353.
33 Watt K, Veldt B, Charlton M: A practical guide to the management of HCV infection following liver transplantation. Am J Transplant 2009;9:1707–1713.
34 Kamar N, Rostaing L, Alric L: Treatment of hepatitis C-virus-related glomerulonephritis. Kidney Int 2006;69:436–439.
35 Rostaing L, Izopet J, Baron E, Duffaut M, Puel J, Durand D: Treatment of chronic hepatitis C with recombinant interferon alpha in kidney transplant recipients. Transplantation 1995;59:1426–1431.
36 Pham HP, Feray C, Samuel D, et al: Effects of ribavirin on hepatitis C-associated nephrotic syndrome in four liver transplant recipients. Kidney Int 1998;54:1311–1319.
37 Sansonno D, De Re V, Lauletta G, Tucci FA, Boiocchi M, Dammacco F: Monoclonal antibody treatment of mixed cryoglobulinemia resistant to interferon alpha with an anti CD-20. Blood 2003;101:3818–3826.
38 Zaja F, De Vita S, Mazzaro C, et al: Efficacy and safety of rituximab in type II cryoglobulinemia. Blood 2003;101:3827–3834.
39 Basse G, Ribes D, Kamar N, et al: Rituximab therapy for de novo mixed cryoglobulinemia in renal transplant patients. Transplantation 2005;80:1560–1564.
40 Bestard O, Cruzado JM, Ercilla G, et al: Rituximab induces regression of hepatitis C virus-related membranoproliferative glomerulonephritis in a renal allograft. Nephrol Dial Transplant 2006;21:2320–2324.

41 Casanovas-Taltavull T, Baliellas C, Benasco C, Serrano TT, Casanova A, Pérez JL, Guerrero L, González MT, Andres E, Gil-Vernet S, Casais LA: Efficacy of interferon for chronic hepatitis C virus-related hepatitis in kidney transplant candidates on hemodialysis: results after transplantation. Am J Gastroenterol 2001;96:1170–1177.

42 Cruzado JM, Casanovas-Taltavull T, Baliellas C, Gil-Vernet S, Grinyó JM: Pretransplant interferon prevents hepatitis C virus associated glomerulonephritis by HCV-RNA clearance. Am J Transplant 2003;3:357–360.

Josep M. Cruzado, MD
Nephrology Department, Hospital de Bellvitge, Feixa Llarga s/n.
L'Hospitalet de Llobregat
ES–08907 Barcelona (Spain)
Tel. +34 93 2607602, E-Mail jmcruzado@bellvitgehospital.cat

Morales JM (ed): Hepatitis C in Renal Disease, Hemodialysis and Transplantation.
Contrib Nephrol. Basel, Karger, 2012, vol 176, pp 117–129

Renal Transplantation from Donors with a Positive Serology for Hepatitis C

Beatriz Domínguez-Gil[a] · Nuria Esforzado[b] · Amado Andrés[c] · Josep M. Campistol[b] · Jose M. Morales[c]

[a]Organización Nacional de Trasplantes, [b]Nephrology Department, Hospital Clinic i Provincial, [c]Nephrology Department, Hospital 12 de Octubre, Madrid, Spain

Abstract

Transplantation of kidneys from donors with a positive serology for hepatitis C virus (HCVD+) remains controversial as made evident by wide variations in practice. Current knowledge derived from unicenter and registry experiences have demonstrated that the use of HCVD+ kidneys in HCV+ recipients seems to be safe in the long-term. This information, summarized in this chapter, has provided the basis for internationally agreed recommendations which limit the use of these kidneys for transplantation in recipients with a positive HCV RNA while on the waiting list and consenting in advance. Avoiding superinfection might require matching donors and recipients based on the involved HCV genotype, an approach limited by obvious time constraints. Because the incidence and prevalence of HCV infection is decreasing and there is a proactive treatment of patients with end-stage renal disease and HCV infection before being included on the waiting list, kidneys from HCVD+ are becoming surplus organs due to the lack of appropriate recipients. The underutilization of these kidneys at a moment of dramatic organ shortage requires organizational measures, including the offer of these kidneys for preemptive transplantation, besides the need of reviewing the evidence driving local criteria.

Organ transplantation benefits about 100,000 patients worldwide every year. Consolidation of this therapy is due to the excellent results achieved with the transplantation of virtually all organs. But transplantation has become a victim of its own success: the number of organs available is unable to cope with the progressive increase in the number of patients included on the waiting list. Figures of shortage reveal that, while at the end of 2009 there were 63,000 patients on the waiting list for an organ in the EU, only 28,000 transplant procedures were performed along that entire year (http://www.ont.es/publicaciones/Documents/Newsletter2010.pdf). A rather similar dramatic situation is described in the US: almost 111,000 patients were registered on the waiting list in May 2011, but the number of transplant procedures performed yearly is about 28,000 (http://optn.transplant.hrsa.gov). As a consequence of shortage, patients might not be included on the lists, especially those with low survival expectancies. Many patients will deteriorate or die while waiting to be transplanted. Added to the unequal distribution of wealth in the world, organ shortage is the root cause for unacceptable practices as organ trafficking and transplant tourism. In this global scenario, governments have been recently called by the World Health Organization to increase organ availability, while decreasing the incidence and prevalence of diseases treatable with transplantation though preventive strategies, in order to progress towards self-sufficiency in transplantation [1].

Different strategies have been devised to increase the availability of organs for transplantation purposes, including the use of organs from expanded criteria and non standard risk donors. A hazard of a decreased graft survival is assumed in the first case and of donor transmitted diseases in the second. Since hepatitis C virus (HCV) infection is transmitted through organ transplantation, donors with a positive serology for HCV (HCVD+) are included in the latest group [2–8]. The transplantation of kidneys from HCVD+ remains controversial, as made evident by wide practice variations. Many centers never accept kidneys from HCVD+ [9]. There are countries with technical and even legal provisions that ban the transplantation of organs from these donors. Finally, the progress made in the therapeutic approach to patients with end-stage renal disease and active HCV infection in recent years, along with the decreased incidence and prevalence of this infection, raise doubts about the usefulness of policies for the transplantation of kidneys from HCVD+. But with demand for transplantation greatly exceeding the supply of donated kidneys, the question to be posed is whether kidneys from these donors should be wasted. This chapter provides an overview of the current knowledge on the safety and efficacy of kidney transplantation with organs from HCVD+, through evidence driven by center- and registry-based studies and summarizes the areas for further research and progress in this particular field.

Transmission of HCV Infection through Kidney Transplantation

Soon after the description of HCV in 1989, several units published their experiences on the transplantation of kidneys from HCV RNA-positive donors, making evident that HCV infection was transmitted through organ transplantation [2–7,10]. Notably, the probability of disease transmission through kidney transplantation was variable, ranging from 14 to 100%, depending on the series. Moreover, the clinical consequences of the transmission of HCV infection for index recipients were also variable. Pereira et al. [4] showed that 50% of the patients acquiring HCV infection through kidney transplantation developed criteria of chronic liver disease (CLD), something otherwise infrequent in the experience of the Columbus University [8]. Variability among the series with regard to the viral load in the transplanted organ, the infectivity of the HCV strain, the volume of the preservation solution, the preservation method used (static storage versus pulsatile perfusion) and the diagnostic tests applied might justify these heterogeneous results.

There was soon a general consensus that kidneys from HCVD+, regardless of HCV RNA, should not be transplanted into recipients with a negative HCV serology (HCVR–). In parallel, the question to be answered was whether these organs could be safely transplanted into HCVR+. Anti-HCV antibodies do not confer immunity and do not indicate an active viremic state. Therefore, the previously mentioned approach would not completely avoid disease transmission. Moreover, superinfection with a different HCV genotype could potentially occur [11]. However, universally discarding kidneys from HCVD+ could be considered unacceptable at a time of organ shortage, particularly in specific countries or geographical areas with a high prevalence of HCV antibodies among organ donors and potential recipients.

Experience with the Transplantation of Kidneys from HCVD+

In March 1990, two Spanish kidney transplant units initiated a pilot experience with the transplantation of kidneys from HCVD+ into HCVR+. First results revealed the short-term safety of this approach. Graft and patient survival among HCVR+ was similar regardless of HCV serology of their donors. A similar percentage of patients in both groups developed biochemical criteria consistent with CLD (ALT levels >2.5 times the upper normal limit during more than 6 consecutive months) [12]. Nonetheless, this policy did not completely prevent the transmission of HCV infection. When HCV RNA was retrospectively assessed in donors and recipients through the polymerase chain reaction technique, five HCV RNA negative recipients were found to be transplanted from donors with a positive HCV RNA. Four of them became HCV RNA positive after transplantation and 2 developed a CLD, as previously defined. As a result of these findings, in March 1993 both Spanish groups modified their policy for transplanting kidneys from HCVD+ by limiting their use to those patients on the waiting list who exhibited a positive HCV RNA before transplantation.

Other unicenter experiences with the same approach as the Spanish one have been published later on with similar short-term results when comparing HCVR+ transplanted with kidneys from HCVD+ versus HCVD– (table 1)

[13–18]. Some of these series highlighted a potential benefit derived from this approach, by demonstrating that time on the waiting list for HCVR+ was significantly shorter for those transplanted with kidneys from HCVD+ [14, 15, 17]. Furthermore, the positive experiences with kidney transplantation from HCVD+ into HCVR+ have been reproduced with liver transplantation also. Testa et al. [19] evaluated the outcomes of HCVR+ of livers from HCVD+ (n = 22) versus HCVD– (n = 115). No significant differences were observed in the rate of HCV recurrence (54.6 vs. 41.7%) or in patient and graft survival at 4 years between the two groups.

In contrast to the positive results obtained in center-based experiences, registry studies have offered contradictory results. By using the United States Renal Data System registry, Abbott et al. [20–22] described a decreased patient survival in kidney recipients transplanted from HCVD+ versus HCVD–, irrespective of HCV serology of the recipient, which became apparent 2 years after transplantation. This suggested the development of an intermediate complication that resulted in a later increased risk of death. The observed higher incidence of posttransplant diabetes mellitus (PTDM) among recipients of kidneys from HCVD+ could be the reason behind it. These data made the authors conclude that caution should be exercised when using organs from HCVD+, and that careful and complete information should be provided to the potential recipient of these organs before transplantation.

What are the reasons for the differences between the results obtained in center-based analysis and those of the United States Renal Data System registry? When taking a careful look at the latest studies, it is important to note that kidneys from HCVD+ had been transplanted into patients with a worse baseline clinical and immunological situation compared to recipients of kidneys from HCVD–. Factors associated with the use of kidneys from HCVD+ were advanced donor and recipient age, African-American race and a high rate of dialysis access complications. These studies also reflected the lack of a specific policy on the use of organs from HCVD+, since they were also used in HCVR–, and there was no information available on the HCV RNA status of the recipients at the time of transplantation.

However, the American registry has been able to demonstrate potential benefits related to the transplantation of HCVD+ kidneys. HCVR+ transplanted with these organs waited 310 days less than the average waiting time for transplantation at their center and 395 days less than their counterparts at the same center who waited for HCVD– kidneys [9]. Most importantly, receiving a kidney from an HCVD+ was independently associated with an improved patient survival compared with remaining on the waiting list for transplantation (adjusted HR 0.76; 95% CI, 0.60–0.96) [23].

Latest evidence on the safety of transplanting kidneys from HCVD+ into HCVR+ has been offered by the Spanish groups piloting the first experiences (table 1) [24]. Information was provided on the long-term outcome (mean follow-up 74.5 months) of 162 HCVR+ transplanted from HCVD+ (group 1) versus 306 HCVR+ transplanted from HCVD– (group 2). No differences were observed in patient survival, and deaths related to liver disease were scarce in both groups (three deaths in group 1 and two deaths in group 2). Graft survival noncensored for death was significantly lower among recipients of HCVD+ kidneys, an observation attributable to the higher donor and recipient age and a more frequent recipient pretransplant viremic state (HCV RNA positive) resulting from the allocation policy applied since 1993. In fact, the negative impact of a positive HCV RNA on posttransplant outcomes of HCVR+ has been described by Mahmoud et al. [25], who showed a higher frequency of chronic allograft nephropathy among HCV RNA-positive recipients. Nevertheless, donor HCV-positive serology was not identified as an independent risk factor for death or graft loss in the multivariate analysis performed in the Spanish experience (table 2). Decompensated CLD (at least one episode of ascites, hepatic encephalopathy and/or gastrointestinal bleeding due to ruptured gastrointestinal varices) occurred in 10.3 versus 6.2% of the patients (p = NS), respectively, in both groups. Donor HCV-positive serology was not an independent risk factor for the evolution towards a situation of advanced liver disease, as previously defined (table 2). Although de novo PTDM occurred more frequently in group 1, HCVD+ was not identified as an independent risk factor either in the multivariate analysis. No differences were observed in the incidence of posttransplant glomerular disease between the two groups.

Limitations of the latest published experience undoubtedly represent research challenges for the future:

(1) Information on HCV RNA among HCVD+ was lacking, but the practice of testing donors with Nucleic Acid Testing has only been recently suggested [26]. However, the knowledge about the HCV RNA status of HCVD+ would not be expected to modify the suggested allocation strategy applied to the use of kidneys from HCVD+.

(2) No information was provided on the HCV genotype of both donors and recipients, which hinders the evaluation of the incidence of superinfection and its clinical implications.

(3) Liver histology was not systematically assessed in this series. Therefore, although no differences were observed between the groups in terms of the clinical evolution of the liver disease, conclusions are not extensive to the histological outcome of the HCV-related liver disease (stable or progressive liver fibrosis).

Suggested Strategies to Decrease HCV Transmission when Transplanting Kidneys from HCVD+

The aforementioned experiences have provided a progressively more solid basis for international guidelines and recommendations for a safer transplantation of

Table 1. Main results of the center-based experiences with the use of kidneys from HCVD+ versus HCVD– in HCVR+

	Ali et al. [13]		Kasprzyk et al. [18]		Mandal et al. [14]	
	D+/R+	D–/R+	D+/R+	D–/R+	D+/R+	D–/R+
Subjects	28	16	60	199	19	10
Follow-up months	36 (12–60)		12–156		15.4 (SD = 2)	
Acute rejection	50%	68%	–		42%	50%
Graft survival	86%		78%	70%	89%	70%
Patient survival	86%		95%	85%	89%	90%
Acute liver dysfunction	16%[1]		–	–	16%[3]	10%[3]
Chronic liver dysfunction	9%[2]				11%[4]	10%[4]
Time on the waiting list months	–	–	–	–	9 (SD = 3)*	29 (SD = 3)*

* $p < 0.05$.
[1] ALT >2.5 times the upper normal limit for more than 2 weeks, but less than 6 months.
[2] ALT >2.5 times the upper normal limit for more than 6 consecutive months.
[3] ALT >2 times the upper normal limit.
[4] ALT >2 times the upper normal limit for more than 3 months.
[5] Decompensated liver disease: at least one episode of ascites, hepatic encephalopathy and/or gastrointestinal bleeding due to ruptured gastrointestinal varices.

kidneys from HCVD+ [26]. A summary of these recommendations is provided below.

HCVD+ Kidneys Should Be Restricted to HCV RNA-Positive Recipients on the Waiting List

As shown by the Spanish groups, the policy of transplanting kidneys from HCVD+ into HCVR+ does not completely prevent the transmission of HCV infection. Therefore, this option should be only offered to those candidates on the waiting list who have a positive HCV RNA and have consented in advance to receive an organ from HCVD+.

The same conclusion is derived from the elegant exercise performed by Natov and Pereira [27] when analyzing the consequences of four different approaches to the use of kidneys from HCVD+. The following assumptions were made:

Morales et al. [24]		Veroux et al. [17]		Woodside et al. [15]	
D+/R+	D–/R+	D+/R+	D–/R+	D+/R+	D–/R+
162	306	28	16	20	20
74.5		23		26.3	34.9
42.1%	37.2%	10%	14.2%	20%	25%
47% (10 year)	58.5% (10 year)	90%	88%	89% (1 year)	79% (1 year)
72.7% (10 year)	76.5% (10 year)	100%	94%	89% (1 year)	94% (1 year)
16.1%[1]	11.6%[1]	–	–	–	–
9.8%[5]	6.2%[5]	–	–	–	–
–	–	9	24	9.9 (SD = 1.8)*	17.8 (SD = 3.3)*

2.4% prevalence of HCV antibodies among deceased donors, second-generation ELISA test with 100% sensitivity and 98% specificity, 100% transmission of infection with the use of kidneys from HCV RNA-positive donors, 20% prevalence of HCV infection among patients under dialysis therapy and absence of clinical consequences of HCV superinfection. No restriction on the use of organs from HCVD+ (all organs used irrespective of HCV serology of the recipients) would be related to 0% of graft losses, but 2.4% of transmission of the infection and 2% of new infections. With a universal restriction on the use of these organs (no organ used irrespective of HCV serology of the recipient), no transmission or new infection would occur, but 4.2% of organs would be lost. By using organs from HCVD+ in HCVR+, 0% of graft losses would occur, but a risk of transmission (2.4%) and new infection (0.5%) would persist. The best balance seemed to be achieved with the restriction of organs from these donors to recipients with a

Table 2. Factors independently associated with patient death, graft loss and decompensated CLD in the multivariate analysis performed in the Spanish experience [24]

	Patient death[1]			Graft loss[1]			Decompensated CLD[2]		
	p	OR	95% CI	p	OR	95% CI	p	OR	95% CI
HCVD+	0.22	0.709	0.412–1.223	0.18	1.248	0.902–1.726	0.92	1.048	0.429–2.560
Donor age	–	–	–	<0.001	1.022	1.012–1.032	–	–	–
Recipient age	<0.001	1.075	1.049–1.102	–	–	–	–	–	–
PRA ≥50%	–	–	–	<0.001	1.912	1.367–2.674	–	–	–
Pretransplant cardiovascular disease	0.05	1.850	0.997–3.432	–	–	–	–	–	–
Delayed graft function	–	–	–	0.03	1.417	1.031–1.949	–	–	–
Acute rejection	–	–	–	<0.001	1.778	1.304–2.425	–	–	–
NODAT	0.003	2.883	1.447–5.746	–	–	–	–	–	–
Moderate CLD[3]	–	–	–	–	–	–	<0.001	9.462	3.887–23.030
Decompen-sated CLD[4]	0.03	2.883	1.447–5.746	–	–	–	–	–	–

NODAT = New-onset diabetes after transplantation.
[1] Cox regression analysis.
[2] Logistic regression analysis.
[3] ALT >2.5 times the upper normal limit for more than 6 consecutive months.
[4] At least one episode of ascites, hepatic encephalopathy and/or gastrointestinal bleeding due to ruptured gastrointestinal varices.

positive HCV RNA before transplantation, with a theoretical occurrence of 2.4% of transmission of HCV infection, but 0% of new infections and no graft losses.

If Possible, the Same HCV Genotype Should Be Present in Both Donor and Recipient

Superinfection with a different HCV genotype could still occur when transplanting HCVD+ kidneys into HCV RNA-positive recipients. Studies in a posttransfusion HCV infection model in chimpanzees demonstrated that a preexisting infection with HCV did not protect from reinfection with a different genotype or even the same viral genotype [28]. Likewise, kidney transplant patients with a baseline HCV infection are not protected from a superinfection with a new HCV genotype [11]. Although mixed infection has not been associated with increased mortality [29], at least one clinical report on a severe liver disease has been published when using a kidney from an HCVD+ into an HCVR+, since donor and recipient were infected by a different HCV genotype (genotype 1 to genotype 2) [30]. Therefore, matching donor and recipient according to the HCV genotype involved would increase the safety of using HCVD+ kidneys, although this strategy is limited by obvious time constraints.

If Available, Pulsatile Perfusion versus Cold Storage Is Recommended for the Preservation of Kidneys from HCVD+

Pulsatile pump perfusion was able to reduce the HCV viral load in HCVD+ kidneys, with the potential of reducing HCV transmission through transplantation [31, 32]. Although these studies have not been reproduced more recently, preserving kidneys through this technique when possible could be recommended for HCV-infected kidneys intended to be used for transplantation.

Kidneys from HCVD+: Surplus Organs?

It has been documented that survival of HCVR+ is significantly better than that of matched patients who remain on the waiting list [33]. Therefore, kidney transplantation is the best therapeutic strategy for patients with HCV infection and end-stage renal disease. However, HCVR+ exhibit worse long-term graft and patient survival rates compared to HCVR– [34]. HCV infection has also been related to the development of posttransplant complications, as de novo PTDM, posttransplant glomerulonephritis, proteinuria and chronic allograft nephropathy after kidney transplantation [35].

The deleterious effect of HCV infection on posttransplant outcomes after transplantation has led to different approaches to the treatment of this infection in patients with end-stage renal disease. Anti-HCV therapy with interferon (IFN) increases the risk of allograft dysfunction, and therefore its use in kidney transplant patients is contraindicated, with the exception of patients developing life-threatening HCV-related complications, as fibrosing cholestatic hepatitis [26, 35]. Therefore, the best strategy is to treat HCV infection in patients on dialysis before transplantation. While in the past, recommendations on end-stage renal disease patients with HCV infection were based on the liver clinical and histological situation, today the negative clinical consequences of HCV infection after kidney transplantation constitute the basis to indicate therapy with IFN, independent of the situation of the liver disease. Benefits of IFN treatment in HCV-infected patients before transplantation in terms of graft and patient survival have not been proven yet. However, they may be related to a decreased incidence of posttransplant HCV-related glomerulonephritis [36]. Also INF therapy in 50 HCV RNA-positive patients significantly decreased the incidence of chronic allograft nephropathy [37].

Treatment of HCV infection before transplantation with the aim of a sustained virological response is obviously not compatible with the policy of using kidneys from HCVD+ in HCVR+. However, the limitations of HCV antiviral therapy should be taken into consideration: a wide range of adverse events has been described with IFN, the rate of non-responding patients is not negligible, the treatment is long, and during this time the patients should be excluded from the waiting list, and it is finally an expensive treatment not universally affordable. Therefore, a group of end-stage renal disease HCV RNA-positive patients will not be candidates for antiviral treatment, some will refuse to be treated, will not respond or withdraw treatment. In spite of having a positive HCV RNA, these patients should be offered the possibility of transplantation, since their evolution will be more favorable than remaining under dialysis [33]. It is in this context where the possibility of being transplanted with an HCVD+ kidney could be offered, with the potential advantage of reducing the time on the waiting list.

The extended treatment of HCV infection before transplantation and universal preventive strategies for HCV infection have fortunately led to a decreased incidence and prevalence of HCV-active infection among patients with end-stage renal disease and therefore among those on the kidney waiting list. Moreover, those HCV-infected patients on the list usually have a long history of renal disease, frequently related to a high immunological risk. In this scenario, it is easy to conclude that HCVD+ kidneys are frequent surplus organs due to the lack of an appropriate recipient. This is even more frequent considering the important variations between centers in their level of acceptation of HCVD+ kidneys. In a recent analysis, Kucirka et al. [9] showed that donated HCVD+ kidneys were 2.60 times more likely to be discarded than HCVD– kidneys. To increase the level of utilization of these organs, organizational approaches are needed that promote their transplantation when these kidneys are not used locally. Moreover, preemptive transplantation of these kidneys into HCVR+ who are not going to receive IFN therapy could be promoted.

Conclusions

The use of kidneys from HCVD+ in HCVR+ seems to be a safe approach in the long-term and a way of using these kidneys that otherwise would be lost. Results provided by center-based experiences show a favorable outcome of HCVR+ in terms of graft survival, patient survival and HCV-related liver disease when transplanted with kidneys from HCVD+. The safety of this approach can be improved by limiting the transplantation of these kidneys to patients with a positive HCV RNA before transplantation and, ideally, by matching donors and recipients according to the HCV genotype. HCVD+ kidneys are being lost today because of remaining doubts that seem to be reasonably overcome and by the lack of appropriate recipients. Organizational measures such as devising preemptive transplantation for HCV RNA-positive recipients accepting to be transplanted with HCVD+ kidneys and international cooperation are essential to avoid the loss of these organs at a moment of dramatic organ shortage.

References

1 WHO, Transplantation Society (TTS), Organización Nacional de Transplantes (ONT): Third WHO Global Consultation on Organ Donation and Transplantation: Striving to Achieve Self-Sufficiency, March 23–25, 2010, Madrid, Spain Transplantation 2011;91(suppl 11):S27–S28.

2 Pereira BJG, Milford EL, Kirkman RL, Levey AS: Transmission of hepatitis C virus by organ transplantation. N Engl J Med 1991;325:454–460.

3 Diethelm AG, Roth D, Ferguson RM, Schiff ER, Hardy MA, Starzl TE, et al: Transmission of HCV by organ transplantation. N Engl J Med 1992;326:410–411.

4 Pereira BJG, Milford EL, Kirkman RL: Prevalence of HCV RNA in hepatitis C antibody-positive cadaver organ donors and their recipients. N Engl J Med 1992;327:910–915.

5 Roth D, Fernandez JA, Babischkin S, De Mattos A, Buck BE, Quan S, et al: Detection of hepatitis C infection among organ donors: evidence for low transmission of disease. Ann Intern Med 1992;117:470–475.

6 Vincenti F, Lake J, Wright T, Kuo G, Weber P, Stempel C: Nontransmission of hepatitis C from cadaver kidney donors to transplant recipients. Transplantation 1993;55:674–675.

7 Aeder MI, Shield CF, Tegtmeier GE, Bayer W, Luger AM, Nelson PW, et al: Incidence and clinical impact of hepatitis C virus (HCV) positive donors in cadaveric transplantation. Transplant Proc 1993;25:1469–1471.

8 Tesi RJ, Waller K, Morgan CJ, Delaney S, Elkhammas EA, Henry ML, et al: Transmission of hepatitis C by kidney transplantation: the risks. Transplantation 1994;57:826–831.

9 Kucirka LM, Singer AL, Ros RL, Montgomery RA, Dagher NN, Segev DL: Underutilization of hepatitis C-positive kidneys for hepatitis C-positive recipients. Am J Transplant 2010;10:1238–1246.

10 Morales JM, Campistol JM: Transplantation in the patient with hepatitis C. J Am Soc Nephrol 2000;11:1343–1353.

11 Widell A, Mansson S, Persson NH, Thysell H, Hermodsson S, Blohme I: Hepatitis C superinfection in hepatitis C virus (HCV) infected patients transplanted with an HCV infected kidney. Transplantation 1995;60:642–647.

12 Morales JM, Campistol JM, Castellano G, Andres A, Colina F, Fuertes A, et al: Transplantation of kidneys from donors with hepatitis C antibody into recipients with pre-transplantation anti-HCV. Kidney Int 1995;47:236–240.

13 Ali MK, Light JA, Barhyte DY, Sasaki TM, Currier CB Jr, Grandas O, et al: Donor hepatitis C virus status does not adversely affect short-term outcomes in HCV+ recipients in renal transplantation. Transplantation 1998;66:1694–1697.

14 Mandal AK, Kraus ES, Samaniego M, Rai R, Humphreys SL, Ratner LE, et al: Shorter waiting times for hepatitis C virus seropositive recipients of cadaveric renal allografts from hepatitis C virus seropositive donors. Clin Transplant 2000;14:391–396.

15 Woodside KJ, Ishihara K, Theisen JE, Early MG, Covert LG, Hunter GC, et al: Use of kidneys from hepatitis C seropositive donors shortens waitlist time but does not alter one-yr outcome. Clin Transplant 2003;17:433–437.

16 Veroux P, Veroux M, Puliatti C, Cappello D, Macarone M, Gagliano M, et al: Kidney transplantation from hepatitis C virus-positive donors into hepatitis C virus-positive recipients: a safe way to expand the donor Pool? Transplant Proc 2005;37:2571–1573.
17 Veroux P, Veroux M, Sparacino V, Giuffrida G, Puliatti C, Macarone M, et al: Kidney transplantation from donors with viral B and C hepatitis. Transplant Proc 2006;38:996–998.
18 Kasprzyk T, Kwiatkowski A, Wszola M, Ostrowski K, Danielewicz R, Domagala P, et al: Long-term results of kidney transplantation from HCV-positive donors. Transplant Proc 2007;39:2701–2703.
19 Testa G, Goldstein RM, Netto G, Abbasoglu O, Brooks BK, Levy MF, et al: Long-term outcome of patients transplanted with livers from hepatitis C-positive donors. Transplantation 1998;65:925–929.
20 Abbott KC, Bucci JR, Matsumoto CS, Swanson SJ, Agodoa LY, Holtzmuller KC, et al: Hepatitis C and renal transplantation in the era of modern immunosuppression. J Am Soc Nephrol 2003;14:2908–2918.
21 Bucci JR, Lentine KL, Agodoa LY, Peters TG, Schnitzler MA, Abbott KC: Outcomes associated with recipient and donor hepatitis C serology status after kidney transplantation in the United States: analysis of the USRDS/UNOS database. Clin Transpl 2004;51–61.
22 Bucci JR, Matsumoto CS, Swanson SJ, Agodoa LY, Holtzmuller KC, Peters TG, Abbott KC: Donor hepatitis C seropositivity: clinical correlates and effect on early graft and patient survival in adult cadaveric kidney transplantation. J Am Soc Nephrol 2002;13:2974–2982.
23 Abbott KC, Lentine KL, Bucci JR, Agodoa LY, Peters TG, Schnitzler MA: The impact of transplantation with deceased donor hepatitis C-positive kidneys on survival in wait-listed long-term dialysis patients. Am J Transplant 2004;4:2032–2037.
24 Morales JM, Campistol JM, Domínguez-Gil B, Andrés A, Esforzado N, Oppenheimer F, Castellano G, Fuertes A, Bruguera M, Praga M: Long-term experience with kidney transplantation from hepatitis C positive donors into hepatitis C positive recipients. Am J Transplant 2010;10:2453–2462.
25 Mahmoud IM, Elhabashi AF, Elsawy E, El-Husseini AA, Sheha GE, Sobh MA: The impact of hepatitis C virus viremia on renal graft and patient survival: a 9-year prospective study. Am J Kidney Dis 2004;43:131–139.
26 Kidney Disease: Improving Global Outcomes. KDIGO clinical practice guidelines for the prevention, diagnosis, evaluation, and treatment of hepatitis C in chronic kidney disease. Kidney Int 2008;73(suppl 109):S1–S99.
27 Natov SN, Pereira BJG: Transmission of viral hepatitis by kidney transplantation: donor evaluation and transplant policies (part 2: hepatitis C virus). Transpl Infect Dis 2002;4:124–131.
28 Farci P, Alter HJ, Govindarajan S, et al: Lack of protective immunity against reinfection with hepatitis C virus. Science 1992;258:135–140.
29 Natov SN, Lau JY, Ruthazer R, Schmid CH, Levey AS, Pereira BJ: Hepatitis C virus genotype does not affect patient survival among renal transplant candidates. The New England Organ Bank Hepatitis C Study Group. Kidney Int 1999;56:700–706.
30 Schussler T, Staffeld-Coit C, Eason J, Nair S: Severe hepatitis C infection in a renal transplant recipient following hepatitis C genotype mismatch transplant. Am J Transplant 2004;4:1375–1378.
31 Roth D, Zucker K, Cirocco R, et al: Transmission of hepatitis C virus by kidney transplantation: impact of perfusion techniques and course of viremia post transplant. Pediatr Nephrol 1995;9(suppl):S29–S34.
32 Zucker K, Cirocco R, Roth D, et al: Depletion of hepatitis C virus from procured kidneys using pulsatile perfusion preservation. Transplantation 1994;57:832–840.
33 Knoll GA, Tankersley MR, Lee JY, Julian BA, Curtis JJ: The impact of renal transplantation on survival in hepatitis C positive end-stage renal disease patients. Am J Kidney Dis 1997;29:606–614.
34 Fabrizi F, Martin P, Dixit V, Bunnapradist S, Dulai G: Hepatitis C virus antibody status and survival after renal transplantation: meta-analysis of observational studies. Am J Transplant 2005;5:1452–1461.

35 Domínguez-Gil B, Morales JM: Transplantation in the patient with hepatitis C. Transpl Int 2009;22:1117–1131.
36 Cruzado JM, Casanovas-Taltabull T, Torras J, Baliellas G, Gil-Vernet S, Grinyo JM: Pretransplant interferon prevents hepatitis C virus-associated glomerulonephritis in renal allografts by HCV-RNA clearance. Am J Transplant 2003;3:357–360.
37 Mahmoud IM, Sobh MA, El-Habashi AF, et al: Interferon therapy in hemodialysis patients with chronic hepatitis C: study of tolerance, efficacy and posttransplantation course. Nephron Clin Pract 2005;100:c133–c139.

Beatriz Domínguez-Gil, MD, PhD
Organización Nacional de Trasplantes
C/ Sinesio Delgado 6, pabellón 3
ES–28029 Madrid (Spain)
Tel. +34 902 300 224, E-Mail bdominguez@mspsi.es

Author Index

Subject Index